THE
EVERYTHING®
RUNNING BOOK
3RD EDITION

MAR – 9 2012
9-13(9) 7-16(13)

Dear Reader,

Believe it or not, I didn't begin running until I was nearly thirty years old. If someone had told me when I was a teenager that I would become a runner—what's more, a marathoner—I would have said he was insane! In high school I couldn't even make it around the quarter-mile track without gasping for air. I started running as part of a lifestyle change, and soon after realized how much I enjoyed my newfound sport.

In 1983, after a year of running, I completed my first 26.2-mile (marathon) race, finishing in 3 hours and 24 minutes (3:24). I've since run twenty marathons in nineteen different states, with a personal best of 3:11. My running experiences have led to a variety of coaching opportunities at the high school and college levels and with the Leukemia and Lymphoma Society's Team in Training program. Through my website, *www.marathontraining.com*, I provide personal training services to runners throughout the United States and the world.

The message I offer to anyone considering beginning a running program is simple: If I can do it, you can too! You'll find that once you start running, your overall health and energy level will improve and you'll experience a more positive outlook on life. Whether you're a beginner training for your first 5K race or an experienced runner trying to improve upon your previous marathon time, *The Everything® Running Book, 3rd Edition* provides comprehensive training information on a wide range of running-related topics. It is your all-in-one training resource—and running companion. Welcome to the wonderful world of running!

Art Liberman

Welcome to the EVERYTHING® Series!

These handy, accessible books give you all you need to tackle a difficult project, gain a new hobby, comprehend a fascinating topic, prepare for an exam, or even brush up on something you learned back in school but have since forgotten.

You can choose to read an Everything® book from cover to cover or just pick out the information you want from our four useful boxes: e-questions, e-facts, e-alerts, and e-ssentials.

We give you everything you need to know on the subject, but throw in a lot of fun stuff along the way, too.

We now have more than 400 Everything® books in print, spanning such wide-ranging categories as weddings, pregnancy, cooking, music instruction, foreign language, crafts, pets, New Age, and so much more. When you're done reading them all, you can finally say you know Everything®!

QUESTION

Answers to
common questions

FACT

Important snippets
of information

ALERT

Urgent
warnings

ESSENTIAL

Quick
handy tips

PUBLISHER Karen Cooper

DIRECTOR OF ACQUISITIONS AND INNOVATION Paula Munier

MANAGING EDITOR, EVERYTHING® SERIES Lisa Laing

COPY CHIEF Casey Ebert

ASSISTANT PRODUCTION EDITOR Melanie Cordova

ACQUISITIONS EDITOR Ross Weisman

ASSOCIATE DEVELOPMENT EDITOR Hillary Thompson

EDITORIAL ASSISTANT Matthew Kane

EVERYTHING® SERIES COVER DESIGNER Erin Alexander

LAYOUT DESIGNERS Erin Dawson, Michelle Roy Kelly, Elisabeth Lariviere, Denise Wallace

Visit the entire Everything® series at *www.everything.com*

THE
EVERYTHING®
RUNNING
BOOK
3RD EDITION

The ultimate guide to injury-free running
for fitness and competition

Art Liberman, founder, MarathonTraining.com
with Randy Brown, DPT, and Eileen Myers, MPH, RD, LDN

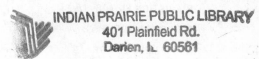
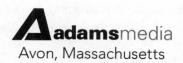
Aadamsmedia
Avon, Massachusetts

This book is dedicated to Dr. George Sheehan and to Dr. Charlie Post. Although they are no longer with us, both inspired me greatly while teaching me so much about the relationship and delicate balance between running and life.

An Everything® Series Book.
Everything® and everything.com® are registered trademarks of F+W Media, Inc.

Published by Adams Media, a division of F+W Media, Inc.
57 Littlefield Street, Avon, MA 02322 U.S.A.
www.adamsmedia.com

ISBN 10: 1-4405-2971-X
ISBN 13: 978-1-4405-2971-9
eISBN 10: 1-4405-3063-7
eISBN 13: 978-1-4405-3063-0

Printed in the United States of America.

10 9 8 7 6 5 4 3 2 1

Library of Congress Cataloging-in-Publication Data
is available from the publisher.

Running Progression on page 128 included courtesy of Vibram, USA, Inc.

The material presented in Chapter 10: ChiRunning® is included courtesy of ChiLiving, Inc.

The information in this book should not be used for diagnosing or treating any health problem. Not all diet and exercise plans suit everyone. You should always consult a trained medical professional before starting a diet, taking any form of medication, or embarking on any fitness or weight-training program. The author and publisher disclaim any liability arising directly or indirectly from the use of this book.

Many of the designations used by manufacturers and sellers to distinguish their products are claimed as trademarks. Where those designations appear in this book and Adams Media was aware of a trademark claim, the designations have been printed with initial capital letters.

This book is available at quantity discounts for bulk purchases.
For information, please call 1-800-289-0963.

Contents

The Top 10 Reasons to Run **x**

Introduction **xi**

01 The Reasons for Running / 1

Striving for Physical Fitness **2**

Getting in the Right Mindset **2**

No More Excuses: Time for the New You **3**

Talk to Other Runners **5**

Benefits of Running **6**

You Will Feel Better, Absolutely! **9**

02 Setting Yourself Up for Success / 11

Finding the Time to Run **12**

Getting Specific about Running Goals **14**

Understand the Effects of Running on Your Body **16**

Choosing and Sticking with a Running Program **16**

Establishing a Foundation **19**

Common Mistakes **22**

03 The Well-Equipped Runner / 25

Running Shoes **26**

The Inside-Out of a Running Shoe **28**

Wearing and Caring for Your Running Shoes **30**

Adding Orthotics **31**

Running Socks **32**

Additional Support Wear **32**

Other Running Necessities **33**

The Runner's Log **35**

04 All about Nutrition / 39

The Nutrition Mindset **40**

The Balanced Diet **40**

Eating Right for Running and Racing **44**

Before, During, and After the Run **46**

What Do "Real" Runners Eat? **51**

Popular Diets **52**

Special Considerations for Female Athletes **53**

05 Time to Get Going! / 57

Starting Out 58

Learning How to Run 60

Stretching Fundamentals 63

The Best Stretches for Runners 64

Working with a Professional 67

Beginning Your Running Program 68

A More Advanced Schedule 71

06 The Mechanics of Running / 73

Running Form Mistakes 74

Style and Mechanics 74

Breathing 75

All about Footstrike 76

It's All about Stride 81

Arms and Hands 83

Posture 84

The Mechanics of Running Hills 85

07 Cross-Training and Weight Training / 87

Cross-Training 88

Ideal Cross-Training Activities 89

Weight Training to Enhance Running 92

Upper Body Versus Lower Body 94

Practical Weight Training 94

Upper Body Exercises 96

Lower Body Exercises 97

Exercises for Abs and Back 98

Weight-Training Tips 99

08 On the Road to Speed / 101

Adding Speed Work 102

Quick Guidelines for Speed Work 104

Hill Repeats 105

Fartlek, or "Speed Play," Workouts 106

Striders and Tempo Runs 107

Interval Workouts 108

Important Warm-Up and Cool-Down Procedures 111

Speed-Work Programs Based on Experience 113

Speed Work for the Experienced Runner 115

09 Barefoot Running / 119

What Is Barefoot Running? 120

Concerns of Safety and Environment 122

Retraining the Barefoot Way 124

How It's Done 125

Injuries and Barefoot Running 129

Running Barefoot . . . in Shoes? 131

10 ChiRunning / 133

What Is ChiRunning? 134

The Elements of Chi (Running!) 136

Making the Adjustments 142

Alternative Applications 144

ChiRunning Versus Barefoot Running 144

11 **Alternative Techniques for Mental and Physical Strength / 147**

Pilates **148**

Yoga **148**

Meditation **153**

Reiki **155**

12 **Injury Prevention / 157**

Avoiding Injury: The Basics **158**

The Impact (Literally!) of Athletic Shoes **159**

Stretching to Prevent Injuries **163**

The Biomechanics of Foot and Leg Problems **164**

Stance and Swing Phases of Gait **166**

Selecting a Sports Physician **167**

13 **Injuries of the Foot and Ankle / 169**

General Injury Guidelines **170**

Achilles Tendonitis **170**

When the Achilles Tendon Ruptures **173**

Ankle Sprains **174**

Anterior Ankle Pain **176**

Athlete's Foot **176**

Plantar Fasciitis and Heel Spurs **177**

Morton's Neuroma Pain **179**

14 **Injuries of the Leg and Other Areas / 181**

Anterior Shin Splints **182**

Dry Heaves or Vomiting **184**

Iliotibial Band Syndrome **185**

Medial Shin Splints—Now Called Medial Tibial Stress Syndrome (MTSS) **186**

Runner's Knee **188**

"Shin Splints" **190**

Side Stitches **190**

15 **Ready for Racing: The 5K / 193**

5K Basics **194**

The Week Before Your 5K **195**

What to Eat and Drink **196**

Physical Preparation **199**

During the Race **200**

After the Race **203**

Themed Races **203**

16 **Completing a 10K and Half-Marathon / 205**

Mileage Buildup for the 10K **206**

Running the 10K **208**

Training for and Running the Half-Marathon **209**

The Long Run **210**

Runners, Take Your Marks, Set, Race! **214**

When the Race Is Over **216**

17 **Are You Ready for the Marathon? / 219**

A Brief History of the Marathon **220**

Factors to Consider When Choosing a Marathon to Enter **220**

Getting Down to Business: The Long Run **222**

Marathon Training Schedules **226**

Mentally Training for the Marathon **229**

Mental Strategies **232**

The Week Before the Marathon **233**

18 **The Marathon Experience / 235**

Physical Preparation **236**

Packing for an Out-of-Town Marathon **236**

Other Travel Considerations **238**

The Final Hours Before the Marathon **239**

During the Marathon **240**

On the Course **243**

After the Marathon **244**

Life After the Marathon **246**

What's Next: Ultra-Running **248**

Ultra-Running Events **249**

Training for Ultra-Runs **249**

19 **Girls (Women!) Just Want to Have Fun / 253**

Comparing Men and Women Runners **254**

Osteoporosis and Menopause **256**

Safety Tips for Women Runners **257**

20 **On the Road All Year / 259**

Running in Cold Weather **260**

Running in Hot Weather **262**

Running Indoors **265**

Using the Treadmill **266**

Shopping for a Treadmill **267**

But It's a Vacation! **269**

Planning for Safety **272**

Racing on the Road **275**

Appendix A: Finding a Running Club, at Home or Abroad **277**

Appendix B: Magazines and Books on Running **278**

Appendix C: Running Online **282**

Index **285**

Acknowledgments

My acknowledgments begin with happy memories of my mom, Sylvia, and brother Jack, who passed away in 1988 and 1995, respectively. They both took the time to listen, care, and exemplify how to live a good life. They also emphasized the importance of giving oneself to others. Thanks also to my father, Sam, and brother Robert, who helped me develop a strong work ethic and passion toward my career and personal interests while demonstrating to me in their own ways how to strive for and attain excellence in all that I undertake.

I owe much gratitude to my first running mentors, the late Dr. Brian Smith and Terry Hamlin, for imparting to me, both as a runner and as a coach, many of the training methods and philosophies that I use today. Thanks also to Randy Brown, my personal friend and fellow coach, for helping me further refine my coaching skills. I have appreciated his counsel and support over the years, and also the material he contributed to this project.

Thanks to all the runners I've had the pleasure to train with and coach over the past twenty-five years, including those with the Leukemia and Lymphoma Society's Team in Training program, members of the cross-country teams at the College of Charleston and North Charleston High School, and visitors/clients of my website, "State of the Art Marathon Training" at *www.marathontraining.com*. You've all taught me more about running and coaching than you can imagine!

Thanks to Eileen Myers, Trace Bonner, Suzanne Goldston, and Carrie Kenedy for their journalistic contributions to this book, along with Ross Weisman for his editorial assistance and support. You all were great!

Enjoy, and I'll see you on the roads!

—ART LIBERMAN

My deepest thanks go to my wife, Fay Mitchell-Brown, who was patient with me throughout this project, and to my daughter Anya who supported me in a way only a four-year-old could. I sincerely thank my friend and coaching colleague Art Liberman for the opportunity to work on this book. I would also like to give my thanks to Noelle Freer and Matt Walsh, two outstanding physical therapists, as well as Danny Dreyer, Hazel Wood, and Georgia Shaw, who were of particular help to me in researching and writing my portion of this book.

—RANDY BROWN
Chico, California

The Top 10 Reasons to Run

1. The number-one reason to take up running is for physical fitness: You'll lower your resting heart rate, strengthen your heart, improve your cardiovascular system, strengthen and tone your muscles, and increase bone density.

2. If you want to lose weight and, more important, body fat, running may help.

3. Runner's high. This is the elevated mood you get when you are running "in the zone" or when you come off a particularly inspiring workout. It's awesome!

4. Running is one of the easiest, most convenient forms of exercise. All you need are the right shoes and clothes, and you're out the door and on your way.

5. Running is a sport that you can do either by yourself or with others. You'll probably want to do both at different times, depending on your mood, fitness level, and schedule.

6. Running alone is a meditative activity. You'll find yourself solving problems that have been pestering you, gaining insight into your life, and just plain feeling better about life.

7. Running with others is a good bonding exercise and can be a friendship-building experience.

8. Running is accessible to almost everyone, from kids to senior citizens.

9. You *and* your dog need more exercise. When both of you start easy and build up, you become a fitness team!

10. Running helps you see the world. No matter where you travel, so long as you have your running shoes and the proper clothes, you can find a place to run. You'll observe things you would never notice any other way, and you'll feel more a part of your locale.

Introduction

WHY RUN? RUNNING IS an exercise available to almost all people. It also has one of the lowest equipment needs of any sport. You don't need a ball, a field, or an umpire. You don't need a gym, a pool, or a track. You might already own everything you need: running shoes, a T-shirt, and a pair of shorts. That's about it.

Sure, there are runners who go beyond the basics. As with other competitive sports, runners make use of gadgets like GPS-enabled sports watches, fancy warm-up suits, and elaborate heart-rate monitors. However, these aren't essential items for the beginner or novice runner.

Another benefit is that you can run alone or with other people. You might run with friends who run at the same pace or run against them competitively. You can choose to run with one person or with a large group. Running is good for the whole family. All ages are encouraged to participate and compete.

There are runners everywhere in the world. Going on a trip? There are runners all over the United States, Europe, Australia, and South America. Just name a locale, and there is sure to be a local running club. Don't know where to go for your next vacation? How about a 5K race in Charleston, South Carolina, or a 5-miler in Chicago? Try a marathon in New York, Boston, Los Angeles, or Hawaii? There are thousands of running events held each year in vacation spots all over the United States and the world, from the 5K to marathons.

The point is that runners are everywhere. And everyone who runs is a runner. Even the man or woman who finishes last in a 5K or a marathon is still called a runner. How fast you run is not a yardstick by which other runners will judge you. In running, it's not you versus the other person. The supreme fascination of running is that it is *you against you!*

Beginning a running program offers numerous benefits, not least of which is your health. For every hour you run 10-minute miles, you burn 4.2 calories per body pound. Jumping rope burns 3.8 calories per body pound and swimming 3.5 calories per body pound. Half an hour spent running is comparable to riding a bike for an hour, chopping wood for an hour, or playing tennis doubles or doing weight training for an hour. Compared with other fitness activities, the benefits of running provide a time-saving advantage in a fast-paced world.

Take it from Ed Daley of Freehold, New Jersey: "I began running in 1979. It enabled me to keep my weight down and it improved my quality of life. I enjoyed life more, I wasn't tired, wasn't heavy. I was able to do more things with ease and comfort. Running improved my fitness and my outlook. I felt better about everything."

In this book you'll learn how to stay on track and become motivated enough to get to the point where you don't want to miss a run. There's also lots of important running-related health and nutritional information as well. Many folks shy away from learning about physical fitness because they think it is complicated, but this book simplifies the subject for you. Your running will benefit from your increased expertise.

Find out for yourself about the new healthier lifestyle that awaits you. It costs pennies a day and will make a huge impact on your life. The latter is the best reason of all to start. Enjoy, and good luck!

CHAPTER 1

The Reasons for Running

As labor-saving advances such as dishwashers, automobiles, and riding mowers have changed people's lifestyles, humans have lost something valuable: regular physical work. Because people have now mechanized even simple activities that use their arms, legs, back, heart, and lungs, their bodies have become correspondingly more flaccid, fat, and weak. People are meant to be active, so much so that their very health depends on it. Running is one way to help your body thrive.

Striving for Physical Fitness

Personal fitness is not a destination that you visit occasionally in life. Rather, fitness is the "journey," an ongoing state of health. Participating regularly in a fitness program ensures your best chance of an improved quality and length of life.

So how do you become fit? As with any project, when you use the right tools the job is much more productive, efficient, and even fun. The tools for fitness include exercise and nutrition. In this book, running is the exercise of choice. But to get started, you need to begin where all activity originates—in the mind.

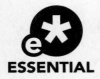

ESSENTIAL

Take a minute to write down five reasons why you want to get fit through incorporating running in your life. You may be surprised by your reasons, which in turn might change over time. Review your answers in one month, then two, to see your progress.

Getting in the Right Mindset

It may seem contradictory, but in fact physical fitness really does begin in the mind. In order for your body to get moving, you need the right mindset. Here are some common reasons people give for *not* running. How many of these have you used yourself?

You Don't Have Enough Time

You might think, "I don't have time to run," or "Running is not the most important thing I need to do today." But you have a choice about how to spend your time. Ask yourself what is the most important thing you need to do today. What is it that you are making time for? How important is your health to you? Keep in mind that of the most effective exercise options, running requires the least amount of time.

You're Worried about How You'll Look

You may also be concerned with how you'll look while running, even worrying that you'll look silly. If you think everyone else who runs looks silly too, at least you'll be in good company! When you're fit and feeling good, though, you won't look or feel silly. Similarly, you might dislike the prospect of sweating a lot when you run. Just remember that sweating is a natural bodily function, and you'll be glad to have a working cooling system.

You Don't Want to Get Hurt

If you're afraid you'll hurt yourself running, read on. When performed properly, running should be neither uncomfortable nor injurious. This book will systematically help you to learn how to run safely so that you achieve a level of fitness that results in a healthier lifestyle. Finally, don't be concerned that you're too old to run. That is the mindset of your old life. Start your new life today. No one is too old to run.

You Don't Want to Spend the Money

Perhaps you are concerned that running is expensive and has hidden costs. However, running is probably the most inexpensive form of exercise. Moreover, being unhealthy is expensive in the long run.

No More Excuses: Time for the New You

There are always excuses for not doing what you really want to do. You probably recognize from the preceding section excuses you've made in the past for not running. Now is the time to stop making excuses. To get yourself ready to be a runner, you need a new way of thinking about running.

Adjust Your Attitude

First, let go of preconceived ideas about fitness and running. Acknowledge and release old negative attitudes. These unhealthy roadblocks are no longer useful to you. You have a choice regarding what you think about, so let those negative thoughts go and start anew.

Maybe you think you will never enjoy running. Think instead about the benefits it provides: new friends, improved energy, a better mood, weight loss, and a healthier lifestyle. As with most new runners who persevere, you will probably come to love running if you just give it a chance.

It is best to approach running with an adventurous spirit. When was the last time you tried something new and healthy? Challenge yourself; be a risk-taker. If nothing else works to motivate you, think of the phrase that Nike made famous: "Just do it!"

Make Time to Run

Think of running as a daily, non-negotiable activity. Do you think about whether or not you are going to brush your teeth each day? Your dental hygiene is a non-negotiable part of your routine that you wouldn't think of not doing. That is how you should begin thinking about running. It is an activity to fit into your day.

Consider time spent running as keeping a health appointment with yourself. If you suffered a life-challenging illness but through regular treatments could reclaim your health, wouldn't you plan your time to go to those appointments? Well, running is a life-saving appointment! It can help prevent a variety of sedentary-based medical conditions, such as cardiovascular disease and diabetes.

Build a Relationship with Running

Becoming a runner takes more than a short-term commitment. Add running to your life as you would build a long-term relationship: day in, day out. Begin slowly, like when two people just start dating. Invest the time to get to know yourself as a runner, and your relationship with running will burgeon.

ALERT

Build a solid relationship with running. You don't start running by doing a marathon. Set as a goal short workouts, and be proud of what you accomplish. Learn by taking small steps, and your relationship with running (or running/walking) will become a lifelong love affair.

Focus on the Health Benefits of Running

Turn your view of health inside out. How much time do you spend tending to your exterior appearance, concerned with clothes, hair, nails, and skin? Many people spend more time attending to their exterior appearance than to their interior health. The truth is, your outer appearance depends on your underlying health. Next time you look in the mirror, look more deeply at your body. Imagine how running will improve both the appearance and inner health of your body. Which looks better—a new piece of clothing or the way your clothes fit after you've lost 5–15 percent of your body fat?

Think of your running time as an investment in your health that yields invaluable returns. With only one half hour a day, you can reap the rewards. You—not other market conditions—control this investment. Regular running is vital to achieving optimal health while also helping to protect you from many preventable diseases. Running costs can be less expensive than what you pay for most life-insurance policies, and you realize the benefits while you are still alive.

ESSENTIAL

"Being an emergency physician, I encounter my share of stressful days (and nights). I have consistently found, however, that I feel better, perform better, and am actually a more empathetic doctor when I work after running. I am convinced of a neuro-hormonal response that takes place in my body and which energizes me, yet at the same time settles me and helps me focus, even under harried circumstances."—Dr. Ben Bobrow, Las Vegas, NV

Talk to Other Runners

If you ask runners how they feel after including regular exercise in their lives, would you expect them to say any of the following?

- Running makes me feel lethargic, grouchy, and stressed.
- Running makes me feel worse about myself.
- Running makes me feel and look terrible in my clothes.

- Running makes me fatter.
- Running makes my sleep pattern poorer.
- Running made me start smoking and drinking.
- Running makes my blood pressure go up.

Of course not! You probably know that people who run regularly claim just the opposite. They boast renewed energy, a better outlook on life, a tendency to eat healthier foods, better quality of sleep, and more. What is it about running that produces such effects? It's the fact that running is a form of aerobic exercise.

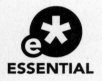

ESSENTIAL

If your friends are runners already, ask them what they like and dislike about running. If they're not runners, ask whether they'd like to be. Recruit one of your non-running friends to start a running program with you and share experiences as you train. You'll double your pleasure as well as be able to share your challenges.

Aerobic exercise does for the body what no other activity can because of a crucial process: the utilization of oxygen. You take in oxygen all the time just by breathing, of course. But when you run, you take in greater amounts of oxygen, and it is delivered more deeply into the body because the heart, lungs, and muscles are working harder. Circulation increases and with it, oxygen delivery. This is beneficial for your body and makes you feel good.

The body loves regular bouts of oxygen-rich exercise and makes accommodations for this. The body actually craves a higher aerobic level. The accommodations are the training benefits that improve the working of the body not only during exercise but also while at rest. No wonder exercise makes us feel better.

Benefits of Running

It is highly motivating to know that you are improving yourself on the inside and the outside. Following are some common and well-documented physiological benefits of running. Let's take a look at what's awaiting you.

Physical Benefits of Running

Running helps to improve respiration, making you an "easy breather." When you run, your body needs more oxygen to fund the activity. Your lungs work harder than when they are at rest to supply the extra demand for oxygen to the body. With repetition over time, your lungs adapt to the extra workload and become more efficient at providing the extra oxygen needed for the activity. The overall effect of this extra work is that you experience more efficient and easier breathing at rest as well as when you are active.

Running also improves cardiac output. Just as success can be measured in terms of productivity, or output, cardiac output refers to the productivity of the heart. It is a measure of heart rate and volume of blood pumped out with each heartbeat. When you run, your heart beats at a much faster rate than when you are at rest so as to provide more blood flow to your muscles. The more you run, the stronger and more efficient your heart becomes. The training effect of running upon cardiac output is such that the heart at rest beats slower, yet is able to deliver larger amounts of blood with each beat. You get more output from less effort, improving your heart's efficiency.

QUESTION

What is meant by the term "training effect"?
Training effect refers to your body's response to a workout. When your body is stressed by exercise, it makes physical adaptations afterward so it won't be as stressed during future workouts. These positive changes that you associate with exercise are the training effects.

As with cardiac output, running also positively affects the vascular system. Blood and oxygen move through the vascular system, the body's highway. As a result of running, veins and arteries become cleaner due to a reduction of fatty deposits. Exercise also increases the number and size of blood vessels, which is the equivalent of more paved streets in your neighborhood, making travel less congested and so less laborious. The effect is to improve your circulation and blood pressure.

An additional benefit of running occurs with improved muscular strength and endurance. When you run, you use one of the body's major tools: its muscles. You need muscular strength and endurance in order to perform activity or work. Muscular endurance means your ability to maintain activity or work over time. One of the effects of running is to keep your muscles functional and strong.

Running also contributes to increased bone density. Muscles are attached to bone, so when you move your muscles during running, it is as if the muscles are massaging and tugging on the bones. The training effect upon your bones has to do with growth. Think of muscular movement like a bone massage that stimulates bone growth. Bone growth helps to keep bones dense, firm, and healthy.

In addition to stimulating bone growth, running can also improve the flexibility of your joints. A joint is the place where bones meet. Movement of your joints feels good; lack of joint movement feels bad. The training effect on your joints from running will improve their mobility.

Another benefit of running you might be unfamiliar with is an improvement in bowel function. Running helps to stimulate the wavelike movement in the bowels called *peristalsis*. This happens in part through pressure changes inside the body as a result of increased breathing. Regular and easy elimination prevents hemorrhoids and constipation.

Another physical benefit of running is enhanced sensory motor skills. As a baby and youngster you learned how to use your sensory skills, you learned about balance and movement in space through activity. In order to keep these sensory skills sharp, you have to use them. A training effect of running is the maintenance and improvement of sensory skills, like balance and movement through space or from place to place.

Psychological Benefits of Running

A well-known training effect of running is the production of endorphins. Endorphins are natural morphine-like hormones that produce a sense of well-being and reduce stress levels. They make you feel good and improve your mood. You may have heard of the "runner's high" associated with long-distance runners, but this group doesn't have exclusive rights to endorphin production. You, too, can produce your own endorphins through regular running exercise.

Another psychological benefit is that running fosters creativity and problem-solving ability in many people. Frequently runners use their daily run as a time to reflect, plan their days, and clear their minds from the pressures of a hectic workday.

ESSENTIAL

"I began running in June of 2000 at a time in my life when I was very depressed and overweight. I knew I had to do something to make my life better. I began running and it changed my life. Since I began running, I have lost fifty-five pounds and my self-esteem and self-confidence levels are very high."—Danielle Utillo, Staten Island, NY

Social Benefits of Running

People are social animals who enjoy and need human interaction. Running builds self-confidence, which spreads to other aspects of your life. Don't be surprised if you feel a bit more outgoing and sociable after beginning your running program; this is another training effect of exercise.

Opportunities for social interaction present themselves indirectly as well as directly. You might directly choose to run with others. But even if you prefer running as a time for yourself, you can still indirectly use the subject as a conversation piece in other social situations.

Your loved ones will be proud of you for your commitment to running. Suppose someone special says to you, "I started a running program a month ago." Do you reply, "Oh no, how could you do such a thing?" or "Oh, I'm so sorry"? Of course not. You probably congratulate him or her and offer support. Others will have the same reaction toward you, helping to reinforce your motivation.

You Will Feel Better, Absolutely!

If you could achieve the psychological benefits discussed in this chapter without exercise, say, through medical and therapeutic services instead, you would have to spend numerous hours and large sums of money, take various medications, and likely deal with some negative side effects. In addition, you would not have much fun in the process, and there are no guarantees that the medical and therapeutic means would work.

ALERT

Everyone begins a fitness program with gusto. But if you do too much too soon, instead of feeling great you could get hurt. Then you'll feel worse than before you started. Are you physically able to start a running program right now? If you're not sure, check with your doctor.

Running can make you feel better with less expense, less stress, and more enjoyment. So now that you have a more positive mindset about running, it's time to learn how to be successful in this new undertaking.

CHAPTER 2

Setting Yourself Up for Success

Before you trot off to create the new you, there are some basic things you need to know to protect yourself over time. After all, this is not going to be just another hobby started and given up; it's going to become part of your lifestyle. The fact that you are reading this book indicates your seriousness about this new sport. Let these pages be your source of information and inspiration as you begin your running program.

Finding the Time to Run

Finding the time to run can oftentimes be the biggest challenge, particularly for those who wish to begin a running program. It seems the busiest people are able to accomplish so much yet still find the time to workout regularly. How do they do it?

It's no secret. Where there's a will, there's a way! Because regular exercisers view health and wellness as one of the top priorities in their lives, something truly valued, they make the time to do it. Even if it means waking up to run at five o'clock! The key to finding time to run is planning ahead. View that time as a non-negotiable appointment with yourself, something to be protected.

Recording all of your professional commitments and personal responsibilities and activities in an organizational planner on a weekly basis is a great way to identify available pockets of time that can be best used to run. Begin by entering in order of their importance those commitments for which you have no control of their time, such as your work schedule, meetings, and appointments. Also include the time you shower, dress, commute, eat, and sleep.

Next, make a list of tasks and activities that don't have to be done at a specific time or may vary from week to week (shopping, laundry, errands). These will be inserted into your planner after you've penned in the time slots when you will train. Keep in mind that the best time of the day to run is when you're most likely to do it!

Research studies indicate that those who exercise early in the morning are more consistent and stick with their programs as compared to people who work out later in the day. Morning is the time when you probably are most rested both physically and mentally. The later in the day you wait to run, the likelihood that unexpected personal or professional obligations will arise, sabotaging your best-laid plans. You may also find that your motivation drops to its lowest level after a stressful or physically demanding workday. On the other hand, there are many runners who can't wait to hit the roads after a busy day, finding it a great way to destress and re-energize.

Don't procrastinate! Insufficient training is a leading cause of injury for those who are new to running and plan to run their first road race. Three or four months may seem like a long time to prepare for a 5K; however, you can't cram for this exam! Mileage needs to be built slowly and consistently to ensure that you will have a safe and enjoyable experience. If you haven't begun training, start now!

Commitment Tools

- **Announce Your Goal**—Whether you simply want to be consistent with your running program or complete your first 5K race, sharing your goal with others and putting it down on paper will reinforce your commitment and make you more accountable.
- **Chart Your Progress**—You will be more likely to maintain your motivation and stick with your training program if you record the miles you've run (along with any other data you wish) in a training log.
- **Just Say "No"**—Depending upon the time you have available to train, there may be occasions when you have to politely decline a social invitation to fit in a run. Don't confuse this with being compulsive, but rather invoking self-discipline as a means to accomplish an important goal.
- **Plan Ahead**—Writing in your planner the day and time you plan to run oftentimes isn't enough, particularly for runners with family responsibilities. Make the necessary arrangements in advance (child care, cooking meals, etc.) to ensure that your workout gets done.
- **Be Flexible**—If you are unable to run as planned due to an unforeseen circumstance, resort to "Plan B." For example, if the babysitter doesn't show up, take the kids to a gym that offers daycare service and run on the treadmill. Or make arrangements to run when your spouse comes home from work.
- **"Just Do It"**—Use Nike's famous catchphrase as a tool in developing the self-discipline and mental toughness to make yourself run, even on those days when your motivation is low. More times than not, after returning from your run, you will be glad you did! Over time, you will discover that working out will be a pleasurable experience that you look forward to doing regularly.

- **Ignore Distractions**—Just prior to the time you plan to run, don't let the computer, TV, or phone grab your attention. Don't let that time you set aside to train slip away.
- **Unforeseen Glitches**—Even the best-laid plans sometimes go awry. If a family emergency or personal illness arises, just resume your training as soon as possible.
- **Mother Nature**—Don't let inclement weather stop you in your tracks. By dressing appropriately, running in the rain or cold can be an exhilarating experience. Also realize that if you're training for a competitive race, the event will go on as scheduled, rain or shine—yet another reason to learn to face the elements.
- **Self-Doubt and Anxiety**—The best way to combat these stressors is to make sure that you get those training runs completed. Knowing that you have trained properly increases self-confidence. Use mental strategies like visualization (seeing yourself in your mind's eye crossing the finish line) and self-talk (telling yourself during times when your motivation to run is low that you will enjoy the race by training properly).
- **Training Partner**—Finding a friend to train with is both fun and motivating. Be sure that her pace closely matches yours. And above all, if she becomes a no-show, run anyway.
- **Reward Yourself**—Treat yourself to a special reward (a new running outfit, a massage, or dinner at a nice restaurant) for accomplishing short-term goals along the way.

Getting Specific about Running Goals

In order to come up with a program that will work best for you, you need to be specific about your needs and goals. Obtain a new notebook and label it simply "Running." On the first page, think about what you want to accomplish. Consider, for example:

- **Is your primary goal to lose a certain amount of weight?** How much do you want to lose? Be realistic about how long it should take. You'll have a sense of how well the running complements the other work you do to reach your weight-loss goal once you are doing it regularly.

Don't assume, however, that a slow mile-long jog every few days is going to drop you from a size 10 to a size 6 in a couple of months. Jogging will certainly help to lose inches, but it'll take time.

- **Is your goal to advance from an occasional run through the neighborhood park to competing in an organized race?** Do you want to start with a 5K, or have you suddenly decided you want to run a marathon next year?

- **Have you chosen running as an economical alternative to a health club membership?** Hey, why not? You're certainly out less money in the long run if in a few months you realize you have neither the time nor inclination for regular exercise. All the same, you won't regret choosing running, both for the cost savings and for the way you're going to feel once you get into it.

- **Do you need to fit running into a very busy schedule?** If so, you may only have time for a half-hour run a day. That's fine! This book will help you to optimize the time you do have.

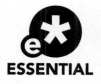

ESSENTIAL

How many times have you intended to change something in your life but it didn't happen? Lots of times, if you're like most people. Well, that's not going to happen this time. You're going to start small, have incremental success, and stay motivated by the growing difference in how you look and feel. You can do this by setting realistic, feel-good goals.

Whatever short- or long-term running goals you have chosen, identify them in your notebook so you can be reminded of them. This will keep you focused when the inevitable temptation to do other things comes up. Don't be vague about your goals. Decide which is your number-one goal, and stick with the program that will help you to achieve it. Haphazardly jumping from one training plan to another will only frustrate you and take you further away from achieving something significant. If possible, find a coach and follow her training plan. A qualified coach will consult with you on a regular basis so that your program can be modified should you experience fatigue, soreness, or injury.

Understand the Effects of Running on Your Body

The outlook of this book is that there's no sport like running to help you feel more fit and focused, physically and mentally. However, after sharing your new enthusiasm for running you might hear excuses from others that it is bad for your joints, that you are too old, or that running is too time-consuming.

You may not want to listen to this advice, but it's important: Running *is* a high-impact sport that does affect people's joints differently. Before you incorporate a running program into, say, the countdown for your wedding because you're convinced it's the only way you'll look and feel great—and keep your sanity—in preparation for the big day, be smart and get a physical exam. The last thing you need is an injury if it turns out that you're not bio-mechanically cut out for this activity.

ALERT

Ask your doctor what she thinks of your starting a running program. You may want to consult a specialist, too, like an orthopedist or someone whose focus is sports injuries. You may need to prepare your body first before you can start running.

Choosing and Sticking with a Running Program

Once you are sure of your primary goal and your doctor has given you a green light, you are ready to choose a running program. Not knowing how to start is often the most significant roadblock keeping people from beginning a running program. With the right guidelines in hand, however, you can get started, know where you are going, and enjoy the journey. The following steps will set you up for success.

Schedule Running in Your Life

Pull out your daily planner or calendar and look at the week ahead. Schedule your exercise session to fit into your busy schedule. Find a desirable time of day or evening to exercise, and make it a regular habit.

Arrange for family cooperation, if necessary. Perhaps your spouse can trade early-morning responsibilities with you; perhaps your children can learn how to make their own breakfast so you can run before taking them to school. When you use your daily planner with an opportunistic eye, you can reserve a small part of your busy day for your exercise time.

Think about ways to include family members if they can't be left alone. Buy a baby jogger or stroller and take your youngster with you. Or allow an older child to ride a bike while you run. A child's designated time for homework can be your designated time for body work.

A frequently asked question is: When is the best time of day to do one's body work—morning, afternoon, or evening? The best answer is: The time when you *will* do it. Some people have a regular schedule that makes it easy for them to plan their exercise at a designated time and day. For others no two days are alike, and they have to create windows of opportunity for exercise time. You manage to make time every day for the appointments you can't miss. You get to work on time, pick the kids up from school, and set aside time to read the newspaper or talk on the phone. You find time for these activities because they are important to you. When you have something important in your life, you are more apt to cherish it and treat it with respect.

Morning running works for a lot of people—all the better if you are a morning person. When you run in the morning you are less likely to skip the workout. You may be more likely to cancel an afternoon or evening workout if you are feeling tired or hungry or if something important comes up. Run in the morning if you can to get the exercise out of the way for the day, and you'll feel better for it. Another advantage of morning workouts is that studies have shown that there are fewer injuries among morning runners than with afternoon and evening runners. This might be because you start slower and warm up longer when you run in the morning.

Schedule your exercise time as you would other important appointments. Give yourself a start time and finish time, and be punctual. A side benefit of setting a regular exercise time is that your partner, boss, children, and coworkers will learn to respect your private exercise time and not to infringe on it unless absolutely necessary.

Make Your Runs Fun and Convenient

Invite a friend, neighbor, or coworker to join you as a regular or even occasional workout partner. Make sure you choose someone whose company you enjoy so that you will look forward to sharing that time. Ideally, find someone who is also a beginner so that both of you will be running at the same approximate pace.

Canine companions are usually happy to be included on jogs. Make sure that if your dog isn't used to running long distances, you take extra care in conditioning him. You have to remember that his paws and cardiovascular system need time to adapt. And make sure your breed of dog is capable of this type of exercise, of course; you won't get far with a Chihuahua or a pug, for example.

ALERT

Remember to carry along some water for your canine runner—dogs can overheat quickly. Check out the dog packs that your four-legged friend can carry on his back, remembering to keep the load light. Also, be considerate of how much running your particular dog can handle.

Wear the Right Clothing

Make your runs more enjoyable by investing in sportswear that gives you confidence. Wearing functional and comfortable clothing can make a world of difference in how you feel working out. If you have been saving your worn-out T-shirts, shorts, and sweats for exercise, think again. Those old clothes may not do much for your motivation, especially if you're a beginner who feels a bit self-conscious about running anyway.

There are many useful fabrics available in the marketplace, such as Coolmax®, Capilene®, and other synthetic-blend fabrics. These are designed not only to look good but also to help keep you cool, reduce if not eliminate chafing, wick away moisture, and make you feel comfortable.

Start Incrementally and Increase Gradually

When first becoming physically active, more is not always better. Before you learned to walk you had to crawl, and the same is true with your fitness regimen. If you want to be successful with your program and feel good both during and after exercise, you need to start incrementally and then increase time and effort gradually.

This is where many people set themselves up to fail. They expect their bodies to perform at levels that are neither realistic nor recommended. Then afterward they wrongly insist that the exercise itself made them feel sore. The point here is to be patient and consistent with your exercise plan.

It is particularly important to start slowly if you have not exercised recently. When you first begin to move, it's as if your body has been in a coma. If someone were coming out of a coma, would you shake her and say, "Hey, come on, get going, faster, harder, more, more"? Of course not. Similarly, when you begin an exercise program, you should be gentle with your body. If you start slowly, your body will respond favorably. To set yourself up for success, start running for small increments of time at low intensity levels until your body has time to adjust to the new activity.

Understanding and applying this pacing of fitness will in fact help you to achieve your goal. Some people feel embarrassed by running at a slow pace at first. You need to put this concern aside so you don't set yourself up for injury.

Establishing a Foundation

Following the basic principles of exercise establishes a solid foundation for a successful exercise program. These principles are centered around the idea that stressing one's muscles at the appropriate level (the workout) followed by rest leads to the next level of fitness. Understanding this important concept can help you determine workout specifics such as frequency, intensity, time, and type. By considering these factors you can optimize your workouts and increase your ability at a safe and healthy pace.

Fitness expert, author, endurance athlete, and exercise physiologist Sally Edwards states in her book, *Heart Zone Training*, "You can only manage what you can measure and monitor." This is certainly true for exercise and health. In order to take an active role in your fitness, keep track in your running notebook of what you do, how much you do, and any other relevant information that relates to your health. Be as descriptive as you like. You do not have to be obsessive about every detail but you should include enough to tell a story about your exercise and health.

The following is an overview of what you need to get started with your running program to train safely and successfully. These topics are explored in depth later in the book, but they're mentioned briefly here as essential matters to take into consideration when first getting started.

FACT

"After having my second baby, I became frustrated that I had not lost the last ten pounds of baby weight. This is when I found Art Liberman's mileage buildup program. I dedicated myself to, and completed, the nineteen-week program. When I finished the ten-mile run, I felt fabulously proud of myself. My self-confidence and self-image soared."—Shelley Barineau, Houston, TX

Equipment and Training Log

Buy a new pair of running shoes from someone knowledgeable. The sales staff in specialty running stores are usually runners themselves. They should have the technical knowledge to put you in the right shoes to meet your biomechanical needs. Don't be afraid to ask questions.

When the mileage total of your shoes approaches 350 miles, it's time to think about purchasing a new pair, particularly if you are above average weight, run on rough terrain, or train in hot, humid conditions. While it's possible for some lighter runners to go beyond 350 miles, the maximum recommended limit for everyone is 500 miles, at which time new shoes need to be purchased. You may think 500 miles sounds like a lot, but as you become a more experienced runner, mileage total will accrue quickly. Training in shoes that have exceeded their lifespan can lead to a variety of overuse injuries that may take days or even weeks to heal properly.

When considering clothing (such as socks, shirts, and shorts), choose those manufactured with synthetic blends that wick away perspiration and reduce the possibility of chafing.

Another item that will improve your running experience is a training log. Use a notebook, calendar, or running log to record the following information at a minimum: miles run, total time run, and shoe model worn. Some runners record everything from the weather conditions to the route they have run to the total shoe mileage.

Keeping a log is important because it provides a history of your running, which is crucial for finding the possible cause of a running injury. Additionally, reviewing a running log helps to determine the training method that has been most effective in turning out one's best performances. Finally, keeping a log is highly motivating, for few runners like to leave too many blank entries. However, do not become compulsive about your running just to "fill in the blanks" or reach a specific weekly mileage total come what may.

There are a variety of websites that provide training logs and show you how to record everything pertaining to your training program, from actual miles run to cumulative shoe mileage. Best of all, most of these sites are free.

ESSENTIAL

A training log may not seem like an essential item in your quest for fitness, but it is. It's a place to set goals, track achievements, and note ups or downs. You'll be thrilled to look back at the mileage you've run, and in turn you'll be more motivated to stick to your plan.

Build a Base

Without question the most important area to focus on when beginning a running program is that of safely building a mileage base, or the distance you run per week. It's essential to start out running in small increments and build on these, no matter how silly or short your distance seems. Never try to take on too much too soon. Doing so can greatly increase your chances of incurring an overuse injury and may ruin your appetite for running.

In a chapter on motivation and success, it's hard not to feel like you can strap on your running shoes and do five miles easily. Although it's admirable to want to seize the day, remember, *slow and steady wins the race*. You'll be running an easy five miles soon enough if you train smart.

In building your mileage base, remember the 10 percent rule: Do not increase either your weekly mileage and/or your long-run mileage by more than 10 percent a week. Doing so greatly increases the chance of incurring an injury, thereby delaying or stopping your training altogether. This is one of the biggest mistakes runners make. Don't do it!

Without a doubt, runners should include supplemental activities such as weight training and cross-training as part of their total fitness program. In particular, incorporating weight training, stretching, and carefully selected cross-training activities into your fitness regimen both reduces the risk of injury and facilitates total body conditioning.

ALERT

You shouldn't even think of training for a marathon (26.2 miles) until meeting certain conditions. Specifically, you should have been running consistently four to five days per week, twenty-five miles per week, for at least a year, without any major injuries.

Nutrition

Nutrition is an essential part of any exercise program. One thing to keep in mind at this point, though, is that nutrition is not just about food; it's about fluids, too. Runners must be well hydrated to run effectively. For runs of up to 60 minutes, water is the drink of choice.

It is also important to emphasize healthy foods in your diet and limit fried and high-fat foods. There is some debate now regarding the proper mix of carbohydrates, proteins, and fats. As a runner you should focus on consuming a mixed diet with carbohydrate foods (grains, fruits, vegetables) filling at least three-quarters of your plate, your protein source filling a quarter of your plate, and a light sprinkle of fats such as oils, butters, or cream.

Common Mistakes

Again, making simple, unintentional mistakes is the most common way for runners to derail their programs. Such runners can be categorized into two major groups. The first type adopts the philosophy that "more is better" and builds his mileage too rapidly, thus suffering breakdown and/or injury.

Individuals in the second group are very inconsistent in their training and may miss several workouts in a row. Then, when they recognize that they are behind in their training, they'll add on additional miles in an effort to catch up. Neither approach will help you to become a successful runner.

Avoiding Injury

One of the greatest challenges of running is to remain injury-free. Although some runners may wear their injuries like a badge of honor, more injuries come from not properly training than from getting hurt on the course. Just as there are different types of runners, there are many types of injuries and treatments.

If you suspect you may have an injury, begin a preventive rehabilitation program to keep the damage to a minimum. Depending on the type of injury, this might mean using ice, over-the-counter anti-inflammatory medication, and above all, resting for a day or two to allow the injury to heal. Should you experience a minor injury while running, apply RICE:

- R = Rest
- I = Ice
- C = Compress
- E = Elevation

If there's swelling or pain, take an anti-inflammatory, such as aspirin or ibuprofen. If your injury doesn't respond to self-treatment in a couple of days, see a doctor.

Stretch Regularly

Beginning runners often underestimate the value of stretching. Stretching is one of the most effective means of avoiding injury and increasing performance and stamina. However, don't stretch a cold muscle before you exercise. It's much safer to stretch after your workout. If a person really wants to stretch beforehand, she should do some brisk walking or a slow 10-minute jog and then stretch. The necessity and benefit of stretching regularly as part of your workout routine cannot be overemphasized.

Utilize Recovery Techniques

There are several therapeutic measures you can take to recover from stressful workouts or from the cumulative effects of hard training over a long period of time. Massage therapy, for example, feels great after a long run, a hard race, and/or weeks of heavy training. Another therapeutic technique is pouring cold water on fatigued legs after a race or long workout. You can also try soaking your legs in a whirlpool of warm water (approximately 105 degrees Fahrenheit) a couple of hours after working out. Something as simple as taking a walk or going for an easy bike ride a couple of hours after a hard workout can also work wonders for tired legs.

CHAPTER 3

The Well-Equipped Runner

Running is one of the least equipment-intensive sports in which you can participate. In fact, all you really need to run are shorts, a shirt, and shoes. But if you're going to do it right, you need to know that not just any shorts, shirts, or shoes will do. Appropriate gear should be comfortable and assist you in staying injury-free. You can have the trendiest gear that money can buy, but if you don't use any of it, so what? Don't get so focused on how you look that you forget that your equipment has to be practical. It has to be easy to care for, easy to take on and off, easy to wash, durable, and comfortable.

Running Shoes

First, you need to outfit your feet with running shoes. These should not be just any running shoes; they should be running shoes that meet your particular biomechanical needs. Take advantage of the fact that running shoes are designed to minimize injury and maximize form and function.

There are three factors to consider in determining the best type of shoe for a particular runner. The first involves what foot type the runner has (high arch, flat foot, or normal arch). It's also important to analyze the runner's footstrike (heel striker, forefoot striker, or midfoot striker) and stride pattern (pronator, supinator, or neutral).

Buying the Right Shoes

To be sure that all of these considerations are met when buying your shoes, you should purchase them at a specialty running store rather than at a wholesale sporting goods store or department store or buying them online. Specialty running stores are places that cater to the needs of runners. Often owned by runners themselves, these stores employ knowledgeable staff who understand shoe construction and are familiar with the latest models and brands on the market. In short, the salespeople of specialty running stores are experts in matching your particular foot type and stride pattern to the specific shoe that will best meet your biomechanical needs.

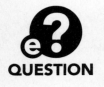

QUESTION

Is there a "best" time of the day to try on running shoes?
To get the best and most comfortable fit for your feet, shop later in the day when your feet have swelled to their maximum size. It is also important to remember that there may be several models of running shoes among various brand names (such as Nike, Saucony, New Balance, Brooks, ASICS, Adidas, etc.) that will meet your biomechanical needs. In other words, don't assume that only one brand will work for you.

When being fit for running shoes, try them on with the style of sock (or one of similar thickness) that you will wear when running. When standing in the shoes, you should have a distance equal to the width of your thumb between your longest toe and the end of the shoe. Ill-fitting shoes without enough room between your longest toe and the front of the toebox can lead to black toenails or toenails that fall off. Additionally, your heels should not slip out of the back of the shoes when you walk or run in them.

Since you will be doing more than just standing in your running shoes, you will want to run around in them before making your purchase. Fortunately, it is becoming more common for specialty running stores to have treadmills on site, which make it convenient to test out shoes you are considering purchasing. For stores without treadmills, run around inside if space permits, getting off the carpet and onto a hard surface. However, don't run outside with them unless you've asked permission first. If the store won't let you try them out, make sure it has a good return policy. Otherwise, shop at another store.

FACT

Base your decision to purchase new running shoes on the number of miles your old pair has on them, not by observing how much tread remains on the outer sole. The midsole of most running shoes compresses and breaks down between 350 and 500 miles, which greatly reduces the shoe's shock-absorption properties.

Types of Running Shoes

Most beginners, as well as people of average to heavy weight, need shoes that provide support, cushioning, and shock absorption. The lighter training shoes (lighter in weight than most running shoes, that is) are designed for experienced runners for fast-paced workouts and races. Some lighter-weight runners can also use these shoes. Because these shoes weigh less than most running shoes, they can help shave a few seconds off one's pace. But due to their lighter weight, they don't offer quite the same degree of protection as a traditional training shoe.

Racing flats are similar to lightweight trainers but are even lighter in weight and thus offer less support or protection. Only the advanced competitor should use them for fast-paced, short-distance training sessions and for shorter races.

When selecting a shoe, remember also that shoe companies work hard to get your attention. Their designs and colors are meant to attract you so that you will buy their shoes. But resist buying a particular style of running shoe because you want to make a fashion statement. You will do yourself a big favor if you think about function over fashion.

The Inside-Out of a Running Shoe

Often when shopping for footwear, you will hear a salesperson use high-tech words to describe the particular features and parts of the running shoe. With a little basic knowledge of running shoes, you can become a more informed buyer and satisfied user. This shoe anatomy session can help you buy the shoe that's right for you.

The *toebox* refers to the toe section of the shoe. It should be roomy enough to comfortably fit your toes. There should be approximately half an inch between your longest toe and the end of the shoe, and half an inch between the top of your longest toe and the top of the toebox.

Next, take a look at shoe laces. You should use laces that are not too long or too slippery. If they are too long, cut them down or use lace locks.

ALERT

Occasionally, runners complain about their feet feeling tingly or numb, particularly during longer training runs. This is sometimes attributed to shoelaces being tied too tightly, which reduces the circulation of blood to one's feet. A simple solution for this annoying problem is to tie your laces just tightly enough that your shoes stay snugly on your feet. Another option that may help is to change the lacing pattern of your shoes.

Held together by the laces is the *upper*, or the material that encloses the foot. Breathable fabrics such as mesh keep feet from overheating in the summer. When choosing a shoe, be sure the upper fits properly; it helps the shoe stabilize the foot.

Beneath the laces you will find the tongue of the shoe. The tongue should be thick enough to protect the top of the foot from the pressure of the laces, but not so long that it rubs against your foot just above the ankle.

At the back of the shoe is the *heel notch*, the slight depression cut into the shoe's heel collar to reduce Achilles tendon irritation and provide a more secure heel fit. The *heel counter* is the rounded place where your heel fits snugly yet comfortably. Too loose a fit can cause blisters on your heels. If you need extra stability (for instance, your feet wobble a lot), look for a stiff heel counter or an external heel counter (a ring that wraps around the outside of the heel). On the bottom of the shoe, look for the *split heel*, a two-part heel structure that separates the outer and inner sides and contributes to a smoother heel-to-toe transition.

Look for heel heights that match your cushioning needs. If you are a big person, chances are you are more of a heel-striker and want more midsole foam under the heel, so you need a greater heel height. Faster runners tend to strike more in the midfoot and need a lower heel.

Getting to Know Your Soles

Most of the cushioning and shock absorption in shoes is provided by the *midsole*, the part of the shoe that you can't see (located above the outer sole). You will want one of two midsole foams: polyurethane or EVA (ethylene vinyl acetate). Polyurethane is denser, heavier, and more durable than EVA. EVA is a softer, cushier material. Generally, heavier runners do well with polyurethane midsoles. EVA is more common because of its lightness and more cushioned feel.

The material that covers the bottom of the shoe is referred to as the outer sole. You will want one of three kinds of outer sole: carbon rubber, blown rubber, or a combination of the two. Carbon rubber is more durable but heavier and stiffer than blown rubber. Some shoes have carbon rubber in the high-wear areas of the rear foot and the cushier blown rubber in the forefoot for a softer feel.

Running shoes also contain stabilizing technology, or devices that reduce overpronation or excessive supination (also called underpronation). These devices are usually in the shoe's midsole on the arch side of the shoe. Some shoes have firmer densities of midsole foam to combat overpronation.

Wearing and Caring for Your Running Shoes

One important aspect to consider in wearing running shoes is how you lace them. Lacing your shoes may sound like a silly thing to discuss, but how you do it can make a tremendous difference in how your feet feel in the shoes. Does your heel slip in your shoes? Does the top of your foot get irritated or fall asleep? If so, the following lacing remedies should help you.

For heel slippage, if your heel moves side to side or up and down, try using the shoe's lace lock. This will bring the heel of the shoe closer to your heel, alleviating the slipping.

FACT

Lace locking to prevent heel slippage is something you can do with any pair of lace-up shoes. To do it, lace normally from the bottom all the way to the next-to-last eyelet. When you bring the lace out of that eyelet, instead of crossing over to the other one, go straight up to the top eyelet and bring the lace through to the back. Do this on both sides of the shoe. Bring the excess lace across and through the small tab you now have at the very top of the shoe, then tie your shoe. This will give you a tight fit at the ankle but not over the rest of your foot.

If the top of your foot falls asleep or gets irritated, you may have a high instep. A high instep causes your foot to take up an excessive amount of space in your shoe. However, if your foot slides around in your shoe and tightening your laces doesn't fix the problem, you may have a narrow foot. In this case, purchase shoes from manufacturers that offer width-sizing options.

Take care of your running shoes, and they will take care of you. It's very important to make sure you keep your shoes in the best possible condition. Worn-out shoes can lead to unwelcome aches and pains or even injury. Follow these tips, and your feet and legs will thank you for it:

• Wear your running shoes only for running—they will last much longer.
• If your shoes become dirty, hand wash them with commercial shoe-care products rather than machine washing and drying them.

- When your running shoes become wet, stick crumpled-up newspaper inside them to accelerate the drying time.

Adding Orthotics

When you think about it, since every foot is unique it's amazing that shoes that fit well and support your movements can be mass-produced to satisfy so many. The truth is, though, that only about one person in four has a normal running pattern. The rest have feet that either roll in too much or not enough when their heels hit the ground. Shoe manufacturers cater to over- and underpronators, but such runners are still more susceptible to injury.

It wasn't too long ago that if you suffered a foot-related injury you had to go to a sports podiatrist and have a pair of prescription orthotics custom made for your feet. Not always an insurance-covered expense, orthotics could cost several hundred dollars. Though definitely worth it for those passionate about running, this solution could be potentially discouraging or even a last straw for those struggling with the sport.

QUESTION

What is an orthotic?
An orthotic is a piece of custom-designed, molded material that is inserted into shoes to compensate for the wearer's biomechanical inefficiencies.

Today, runners can try to reduce injury as a result of their imperfect strides by supplementing their running shoes with over-the-counter, orthotic-like arch supports, such as Superfeet®. Certainly superior to foam-cushioned insoles, these inserts are designed to provide shock absorption while compensating for pronation and other irregularities. It's important to speak with someone knowledgeable about biomechanics and running shoes before simply ditching the sock liner of your new shoes and putting in an over-the-counter orthotic you think will help. In fact, without proper understanding of its purpose, your use of an orthotic may *increase* your risk of injury.

Running Socks

Some people tend to take socks for granted, but it only takes one blister to bring your feet to your attention. A general rule in choosing socks is that activities that produce a lot of foot friction require a thicker sock. For example, sports like basketball and racquetball generate a lot of friction and warrant thicker socks. Unless you are running on trails (which can create high friction), you can be comfortable running in a thin sock, but again, go with what feels good to you.

Steer clear of socks made from 100 percent cotton as these will not wick away perspiration or moisture, increasing your chances of getting blisters. There are numerous synthetic fabrics being used today that make socks fit, hold up, and wick away moisture better than ever before (so that you don't have wet feet, which can cause blisters). Look for synthetic blends like those made from polyester, acrylic, or Coolmax®, which are best at wicking away moisture. There is also no need to suffer with socks that bunch and slip down into your shoes. These will only irritate you while running and may produce some nasty blisters.

Additional Support Wear

In addition to shoes and socks, you may be in need of additional support wear for your body. Running creates a lot of movement and vibration of the body that can cause discomfort. Fortunately, there are many products on the market to aid both men and women in exercise comfort.

Athletic Supporters, Jock Straps, and Compression Shorts

Personal preference dictates the use of these invaluable protective and supportive devices for boys and men. For contact activities (martial arts) and even some unintentional contact sports (soccer), athletic cups and supporters may be preferred. Neither of these is really necessary for running. However, support for men is still a big issue. Two garment styles that have taken the place of more traditional supporters are running shorts with built-in liners and compression shorts. They reduce movement and vibration, which leads to greater comfort.

Sports Bras

Unlike male support mechanisms that have been around a long time, sports bras were first introduced in the late 1970s. They didn't become widely accepted until the 1980s, when the real running boom hit.

There are three types of sports bras: compression, encapsulation, and combination. Compression-style bras use the pressure of the fabric to squeeze or press the breasts flat against the chest, limiting movement. Small- to medium-breasted women often favor this style. The encapsulation style limits movement by surrounding and supporting the breasts with reinforced seams or wire (like an underwire bra). Larger-breasted women typically prefer this style. The combination style combines compression and encapsulation.

Other Running Necessities

Depending on the weather and how comfortable you'll be wearing them, you might want to run with one or more of the following: sunglasses, a sweatband, a baseball cap, a wool hat, gloves, and a key/change carrier that can be wrapped around your wrist, ankle, or waist. You can get as low-tech or high-tech as you want, now that there are materials that reflect or absorb light, wick moisture away from your skin, insulate while remaining lightweight and dry, and so on. If you run at night, you'll need reflective gear (or you can sew or glue reflective tape to your gear). Also, don't forget sunscreen when you're out during the day. You'll need it in the winter as much as in the summer.

A Running Watch

You will come to depend on your running watch the way you depend on your wristwatch when you think you might be late for work. Your running watch will let you know how you're doing at all times.

The watch you use doesn't have to be expensive. Before purchasing a watch for running, decide what functions you think you'll really use. Most digital chronograph watches include a stopwatch, an alarm, lap settings (also called split timing), a glow light for seeing your time at night, and a regular clock. The stopwatch will be the part you use most, so make sure it's easy to start, stop, and reset, and is also waterproof.

But why simply monitor your overall time and distance when you can learn so much more about your performance during a run? There are a variety of GPS-enabled sports watches that allow you to continuously monitor your speed, distance, pace, calories burned, and heart rate throughout the various phases of your workout. You can even make your workouts more challenging with a virtual partner feature, enabling you to train alongside a digital competitor with programmable specified time, distance, and pace goals. Some devices feature the capability of downloading information to a computer so you can both store the data and keep an online running log. Some of the more popular sports watch brands include Garmin, Polar, and Timex.

Water, Water Anywhere

Although a runner's best friend in the short run is drinking water, workouts longer than 60 minutes additionally require a consumption of sports drinks—critical both for keeping heat-driven illness at bay as well as for ensuring optimal performance. Thankfully, today there are now practical and convenient carrying systems available that you can strap onto your waist and that hold a variety of plastic bottle sizes. Other systems strap to your back and include fluid delivery tubes, making sipping easy and convenient so you can access water at all times.

Jog to the Music

Some runners consider the gear they use to listen to music while they run as important as their clothes, watch, or even fluids. With portable music systems getting increasingly smaller and lighter, it is infinitely easier and more comfortable to get into the groove with your favorite selection of Motown, funk, classic rock, classical music, or even talk radio than ever before. Runners compare and contrast playlists on their iPods as frequently as they do split times or which races are their favorites. Like chatting with a running buddy, listening to music can make a run feel less challenging and shorter—and who doesn't appreciate that? Runners who use portable music-playing systems need to be especially mindful of their surroundings, however.

The Runner's Log

How does a training log qualify as equipment? Because without a training log, you're running in the dark. There are three main reasons for keeping a log. First, it provides a history of your running, crucial to finding a possible cause of a running injury. Second, reviewing a running log helps determine which training methods have been most effective in prompting one's best performances. Finally, keeping a log is highly motivating, since few runners like to leave too many empty lines. (See Table 3-1 for a sample log.) Additionally, it's useful to keep a shoe mileage chart (see Table 3-2), which makes it easy to determine when it's time to purchase a new pair of shoes (when your shoes reach an upper limit of 350–500 miles).

What to Log

At a minimum you need to record the distance you have actually covered in your workout. This total should also include your warm-up and cool-down mileage because, after all, you did cover that distance on foot.

You should estimate your average pace per mile running by time rather than by mileage. To do this, you can visit a track and run four laps at a relaxed pace; four times around most high school or college tracks equals 1,600 meters, or very close to a mile (0.9942 miles). Then run for a specific amount of time and determine the mileage covered. For example, if your easy pace for a mile is 9 minutes, run for a little over 36 minutes, and call the workout a 4-miler.

The next item to log is the time duration of your workout. In other words, determine how many total minutes you were moving and running, walking, or a combination of both. If you are using the run/walk method of training, you can be even more specific if you like by recording the actual minutes you were running and the minutes you were walking.

▼ TABLE 3-1: RUNNER'S LOG

Week of:		Sun.	Mon.	Tues.	Wed.	Thurs.	Fri.	Sat.	Total
___/___ to ___/___	Time								
	Mileage								
___/___ to ___/___	Time								
	Mileage								
___/___ to ___/___	Time								
	Mileage								
___/___ to ___/___	Time								
	Mileage								
___/___ to ___/___	Time								
	Mileage								
___/___ to ___/___	Time								
	Mileage								
___/___ to ___/___	Time								
	Mileage								
___/___ to ___/___	Time								
	Mileage								
___/___ to ___/___	Time								
	Mileage								
___/___ to ___/___	Time								
	Mileage								

▼ **TABLE 3-2: SHOE MILEAGE CHART**

Pair #1 _____			Pair #2 _____			Pair #3 _____		
Date	DM	CM	Date	DM	CM	Date	DM	CM
Date	DM	CM	Date	DM	CM	Date	DM	CM
Date	DM	CM	Date	DM	CM	Date	DM	CM
Date	DM	CM	Date	DM	CM	Date	DM	CM
Date	DM	CM	Date	DM	CM	Date	DM	CM
Date	DM	CM	Date	DM	CM	Date	DM	CM
Date	DM	CM	Date	DM	CM	Date	DM	CM
Date	DM	CM	Date	DM	CM	Date	DM	CM
Date	DM	CM	Date	DM	CM	Date	DM	CM
Date	DM	CM	Date	DM	CM	Date	DM	CM
Date	DM	CM	Date	DM	CM	Date	DM	CM
Date	DM	CM	Date	DM	CM	Date	DM	CM
Date	DM	CM	Date	DM	CM	Date	DM	CM
Date	DM	CM	Date	DM	CM	Date	DM	CM
Date	DM	CM	Date	DM	CM	Date	DM	CM
Date	DM	CM	Date	DM	CM	Date	DM	CM
Date	DM	CM	Date	DM	CM	Date	DM	CM
Date	DM	CM	Date	DM	CM	Date	DM	CM
Date	DM	CM	Date	DM	CM	Date	DM	CM
Date	DM	CM	Date	DM	CM	Date	DM	CM
Date	DM	CM	Date	DM	CM	Date	DM	CM
Date	DM	CM	Date	DM	CM	Date	DM	CM

Key: DM = Daily Mileage; CM = Cumulative Mileage

For runners who rotate two or more pairs of running shoes for their training from day to day, or even if you own just one pair, it's also important to write down the shoe model you used for your workout and the respective miles run in that particular shoe. This will enable you to track its wear. Many injuries can be traced to training shoes that are worn out.

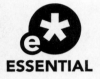

ESSENTIAL

To log your information you can use a blank calendar or a spiral notebook. *Runner's World* also produces a comprehensive training log that you can use to record your workouts for an entire year. There are also a variety of free websites that enable you to record the specifics of your workout (mileage, shoes, duration, etc.). In short, the choice is yours.

Other indicators you can record include, but are not limited to: heart rate (for those runners who use a monitor before and during exercise), weather (temperature, wind, conditions), the specific route you ran, how your legs felt during and after the workout, other cross-training activities done that day, what you had to eat, how much water you took in, and so on. Some runners record their heart rate (pulse) at bedtime and upon awakening in the morning to determine if they are overtraining. The key is to have a program of what you are willing to record on a day-by-day basis.

Using a Calendar

Another way to keep a log is by using a calendar. This can sometimes be better than a separate log because you can also use it to record other events in your life. This gives you an understanding of how other events can be distractions or hindrances to your running. One drawback to calendars is that they are not always easy to write on and don't offer the space to write more extensive notations. Even so, calendars are easy to maintain and give you the opportunity to make running part of your everyday life.

CHAPTER 4

All about Nutrition

Whether your goal is to run short-distance, long-distance, or all distances, your nutritional intake is key to both how well you will perform and how well you will feel before, during, and after a run. The information in this chapter is your guide to what and how to eat in order to feel your best and to perform your best in runs and races. It will also describe some of the popular diets for runners along with special considerations for female runners.

The Nutrition Mindset

Do you have the nutrition mindset? Do you think about what, when, and how you eat? Do you have focus to optimize your diet to fuel your muscles to operate efficiently every day? The nutrition mindset starts with understanding how the body wants to be fed while at rest and with activity. It is about understanding the value of the different foods that are available to you and choosing the right balance and right amounts at the right times every day.

According to the Merriam Webster definition, *nutrition* is the act or process of nourishing or being nourished; specifically, the sum of the processes by which an animal or plant takes in and utilizes food substances. You eat to fuel every organ of your body for energy and function.

The nutrition mindset is eating for health and performance each and every day—not just before a race. When you eat a healthy diet each and every day, you fuel your muscles and organs with protective nutrients that are the foundation of optimal performance, good health, and feeling great!

The Balanced Diet

On June 2, 2011, the U.S. Department of Agriculture released the new food group guidance system called "Choose MyPlate" (*www.choosemyplate.gov*). The plate replaces the pyramid to help Americans implement healthy eating habits. MyPlate follows the 2010 Dietary Guidelines for Americans, suggesting that you fill half of your plate with fruits and vegetables and fill the other half with whole grains and a source of lean protein. Along with this plate of food is a side serving of a low-fat or nonfat dairy product. Foods and ingredients to use only sparingly consist of saturated fats, sodium, added sugars, and alcohol.

For the first time the picture of a balanced diet should make sense because you can visually see it just as you do when we eat it—on a plate, rather than listed on a pyramid. Along with the picture of a balanced meal, the dietary guidelines suggest you eat what you like and take time to eat to truly enjoy the meal. Eating too fast, eating on the go, and grazing mindlessly may cause you to eat too many calories. Even as a runner, it can be helpful to use smaller-sized plates, bowls, and glasses to help you control portions. Even a runner might overeat more than the body needs simply because the food was right in front of you and not because your body was necessarily hungry for it.

QUESTION

What is a calorie?
Technically, a food calorie is a unit of energy—the amount of energy necessary to raise the temperature of one kilogram of water by 1 degree Celsius. The number of calories in a food portion tells us how much energy a food potentially gives the body. If this energy is not used by the body, it typically is stored in the body as fat for later use. Calories are used to fuel the body, including the heart, lungs, brain, and skeletal muscle. The number of calories we need varies based on our age, gender, size, health, and activity level.

A balanced diet means more than just one plate of food that meets diverse nutritional needs. It means eating this plate of food or a mini-plate of this food regularly spaced throughout the day, starting with first thing in the morning (breakfast). Given that the goal is to eat moderate amounts each time you eat, it is likely that you may be consuming a plate or mini-plate of food anywhere from three to six times a day.

Let's break this plate down further to best understand the nutrients you need for running. There are six nutrients needed to sustain life—water, carbohydrates, proteins, fats, vitamins, and minerals.

Water

Water is the most important nutrient for the body. Your body consists of 60–70 percent water, and without water you would die. Water is responsible for transporting other nutrients to your muscles and excreting wastes through the kidneys and other organs for disposal. Water lubricates joints and helps cushion the body's organs. Water helps regulate your body temperature. Water also is essential for maintaining healthy skin.

Carbohydrates

The primary function of carbohydrates is to provide energy to the body, especially the energy for brain and nervous system functioning. Carbohydrates also provide energy to the muscles needed in activity. Foods containing carbohydrates are categorized as complex and simple carbohydrates. Complex carbohydrates are typically referred to as starches. They are formed when sugars link together to form a complex chain of sugar molecules. Potatoes, rice, pasta, breads, legumes, and other starchy vegetables are referred to as complex carbohydrates. Simple carbohydrates are sugars such as table sugar, corn syrup, honey, and even milk sugar as well as fruit, fruit juice, and some vegetables. Simple carbohydrates are made of either single or double sugar molecules that are quickly absorbed into the bloodstream. Other examples of simple carbohydrates are candy, sugar-sweetened beverages, syrups, and most sports drinks and gels.

FACT

Dietary fiber is the nondigestible portion of fruits, vegetables, and grains. Fiber has many benefits such as promoting normal bowel movements, regulating blood sugar, lowering cholesterol, and reducing risk of certain cancers. Fiber holds water as it moves through the digestives system. Make sure you drink enough fluid when consuming a high-fiber diet.

Carbohydrates can also be classified by how fast they are absorbed. Quick-absorbing carbohydrates raise blood sugar levels quickly. These carbohydrates are good recovery carbohydrates after a run. Examples of quick-absorbing carbohydrates include baked potatoes, honey, white bread, and refined cereal. Slow carbohydrates are digested more slowly and cause a more gradual rise in blood sugar. These slow-absorbing carbohydrates are more sustaining and are best consumed before exercise for sustained energy. Examples of slow-absorbing carbohydrates include apples, apricots, oatmeal, and dried beans.

Protein

Proteins are the building blocks of muscle and are present in every cell of the body, including organs, hair, and skin. Protein is made from amino acids. There are eight essential amino acids necessary to form the protein found in muscle, organs, hormones, and enzymes. These eight amino acids must come from your diet since your body can't make them. Food sources of protein that contain all essential amino acids include meat, fish, poultry, eggs, dairy, and soybeans. Grains and other plant foods do not contain all of the essential amino acids and must be combined with other foods containing the missing amino acids to form a complete protein.

Fat

Fat is a nutrient that is a part of every cell membrane. Fat contains essential fatty acids needed for hormone production. Fat in the diet allows fat-soluble vitamins (vitamins A, D, E, and K) to be absorbed into the body. Fat is often misunderstood because fat has been associated with heart disease. Through decades of research we now understand that monounsaturated and polyunsaturated fats are protective and important in a healthy diet, while saturated fats are harmful to our health. Examples of monounsaturated fats are olive oil, canola oil, and nuts. Polyunsaturated fats consist of corn oil, soy oil, and fatty fish. Examples of saturated fat are butter, cream, cheese, and meat fat. Consuming lean meats and low-fat dairy are helpful ways to limit saturated fat.

ALERT

Hydrogenated fats are processed fats that act similar to saturated fats. Hydrogenation is the process of adding hydrogen to polyunsaturated fats to give food a longer shelf life and to add flavor. Baked goods such as cookies and crackers, margarines, and certain peanut butters contain hydrogenated or partially hydrogenated fats.

Vitamins and Minerals

Both vitamins and minerals are necessary for life. The body cannot make vitamins and minerals. Vitamins are sometimes referred to as the "sparkplugs" of our diet—vitamins are effective in allowing our body to release energy but they contain no energy value in and of themselves. Minerals support vital processes such as oxygenation of the blood, heart rhythm, and bone structure. The best way to consume vitamins and minerals is through a wholesome, balanced diet.

Eating Right for Running and Racing

The basics of eating for running and racing are similar to the guidelines found at ChooseMyPlate.gov. The diet composition for a runner consists of eating mostly carbohydrates, a moderate amount of protein, and limited fat. Eating right for running and racing requires hydrating adequately and consuming sufficient fuel for your muscles.

Hydrate Adequately

The single biggest reason for poor running performance and early fatigue is related to poor hydration. Dehydration impacts running performance when you lose just 2 percent of your body weight in water. Choosing mostly water along with fruits, fruit juices, and dairy drinks throughout the day aids in keeping you well hydrated. As soon as you are dehydrated, your heart needs to work harder, your body temperature elevates, and you start to feel sick. Under nonathletic conditions, the rule of thumb is to drink eight 8-ounce glasses of fluid per day, which protects most people from becoming dehydrated. With physical activity, the amount you need to drink increases. Unfortunately, during exercise, the body's thirst mechanism might not be a good guide. Instead of relying totally on thirst, it may be helpful to use your sweat rate and the clock to guide you in consuming adequate fluids.

Calculating Sweat Rate

Your sweat rate will vary by climate conditions. When calculating your sweat rate, run your normal running pace for 1 hour in a variety of temperatures and humidity conditions. Complete the following steps.

- **Step one:** Take your weight in the nude before and after a run and note the difference in ounces.
- **Step two:** Add to this difference the amount of fluid you drank during the run.
- **Step three:** Take this amount and divide by 4 to determine how much you should drink every 15 minutes.

▼ **EXAMPLE**

Weight before: 200 pounds
Weight after: 199 pounds
Drank: 8 ounces of water
Sweat loss: 24 ounces/hour

Divide your hourly fluid loss by 4 = 6 ounces every 15 minutes.

FACT

It was once thought that caffeinated beverages dehydrated rather than hydrated the body. Recent studies have shown that caffeine in most popular beverages does not keep the body from absorbing fluid, and caffeinated drinks are acceptable to count as fluid intake. Caffeinated beverages, however, should not be used as the exclusive hydrating beverage.

If your weight after a run is greater than your weight before the run, you may be drinking too much during the run. Your post-run weight should be the same or within 1 to 2 pounds less than your pre-run weight.

For runs lasting over 1 hour, it is recommended that your fluid consist of a sports drink that provides carbohydrates, fluids, and sodium. The carbohydrates help prevent your using up your muscle glycogen, the fluid keeps you hydrated, and the sodium keeps your electrolytes in balance. (Electrolytes are chemicals in the body that carry electrical charges necessary for cell function and for using caloric energy.)

Adequate Fuel

When you are running, your body relies on stored carbohydrates and fats to give you energy. Even the leanest runner has sufficient fat stores for running, and yet when you run out of carbohydrate stores, you "hit the wall." Carbohydrates are stored in your muscles and your liver in the form of glycogen, which breaks down into sugar for use as energy. Adequate glycogen levels are key to a successful run. Glycogen capacity improves through a combination of a diet adequate in carbohydrates, and through training. Both diet and training optimize the amount of glycogen that the muscles can store.

Viewing ChooseMyPlate.gov, you see that three-quarters of the plate is made up of carbohydrates foods (fruits, vegetables, and grains), which equals about 50 percent of your caloric intake from carbohydrates. Look at your own "plate of food" to evaluate if you have enough carbohydrates. Fruits, starchy vegetables such as beans, peas, potatoes, and corn, along with breads and cereals, are higher in carbohydrate content per serving than non-starchy "green" vegetables. When evaluating your meal, make sure it is not comprised of exclusively green salad ingredients or you will not be consuming enough carbohydrates.

Before, During, and After the Run

How you fuel your body before, during, and after the run makes a difference in how you feel and how you perform.

Before Your Run

Follow these guidelines as you prepare for your workout.

Hydrating Before the Run

As was mentioned previously, if you start your run fully hydrated you'll have more success. A rule of thumb is to consume 14–20 ounces of water or sports drink 2–3 hours before you run. Drink 8 ounces right before you start your run. The best way to know if you are drinking enough is to note the color of your urine. If darker than a pale yellow, you need more fluid; if your urine is completely clear, you may be drinking too much before your run.

Fueling Before the Run

The amount you eat before a run will vary by the timing of your run. A moderate-sized meal is optimally consumed 3–4 hours before a run. If there are only 2 hours between your meal and your run, the portion should be smaller. If you are short on time before your run, you'll only have room for a snack. The point is to have your food fully digested before you run so that the fuel you just consumed provides energy for your working muscles. Your pre-run meal should consist of the components of a balanced meal while minimizing fat and fiber to minimize digestive distress. Liquid meals may be better tolerated when your food is consumed closer to the run. The small amount of protein in your pre-run meal helps build and repair muscle tissue and may help with post-exercise soreness. Pre-run food examples include a peanut butter and jelly sandwich, a fruit smoothie, or a turkey and cheese sandwich.

ALERT

A small percentage of runners may experience rebound hypoglycemia when consuming a sugary snack 30–60 minutes before running. Symptoms may include weakness, lightheadedness, trembling, and heart palpitations during the run. Solutions include using a slow-absorbing carbohydrate fuel source as your snack, or better yet, being prepared by having regularly spaced meals and snacks 1–2 hours before the run.

Frequently Asked Questions

I just woke up out of bed and go right out the door for my run. How can I eat?

> If you just woke up you can be sure your glycogen stores are lower than optimal. If you don't have that much time before your run, consume at least 8 ounces of a liquid carbohydrate drink before taking your first steps.

Eating before I run gives me GI distress.

> If you can't eat anything before your morning run, make sure the evening-before meal was sufficient. It may also help to consume a mini-meal before bedtime. Do make sure you consume water before starting your run. Also, some people can't eat before a run but can eat without GI distress during the run. Have a carbohydrate source of fuel with you during the run.

I run right after work and I'm already starving.

> When you run after work, make sure you have available a midafternoon snack sufficient in carbohydrates but with some protein to hold you through the afternoon. When you get too hungry, you are more apt to reach for a high-fat food source right before your run, giving you an upset stomach during or after the run.

During the Run

You should use the following instructions during your workouts.

Hydrating During the Run

For any run lasting more than 20 minutes, hydration during the run is important. In cool conditions you may not need to hydrate during a run lasting 30–45 minutes. But if the heat and/or humidity is elevated, don't trust your thirst. The American College of Sports Medicine recommends that athletes consume fluids at a rate close to their sweat rate, which for most is 3–7 ounces every 15 minutes.

Fueling During the Run

Fuel your body with 30–60 grams of a fast-absorbing carbohydrate for every hour of your run. Ideally this is broken down into 10–20 grams of carbohydrate every 20 minutes. Your fuel can be in the form of a carbohydrate-based beverage, gels, jellybeans, fruit, or carbohydrate snack bar, based on your preference and tolerance. Experiment with sports drinks and bars during your training runs to find out what works best for you. Fueling during the run can consist of sports drinks, fruit slices, gels, gummy chews, or bites of low-fat sports or granola bars.

FACT

Optimal carbohydrate concentration in a sports drink should be 4–8 percent concentration, or 10–18 grams per 8 ounces. Best carbohydrate sources include a combination of glucose, maltodextrin, sucrose, and dextrose. Sports drinks that contain only electrolytes are insufficient for runs lasting longer than 45 minutes unless another carbohydrate source, such as gels, bars, chews, or fruit, is ingested.

Consider This

I drink lots of water during my 2-hour runs but I don't eat. Is there a problem with that?

> Running long distance and only consuming water can lead to a condition called *hyponatremia*. Hyponatremia is a condition where there is too little sodium in the bloodstream. Sodium is lost through sweat, and plain water consumed in excess during a run dilutes the sodium balance. Even when well acclimated, it is always a good idea to use endurance drinks that contain adequate sodium as well as needed carbohydrates.

After the Run

Follow these tips to ensure a safe recovery after you've finished your run.

Hydrating After the Run

Continue to drink fluids after your run is complete. Pay attention to your urge to urinate and note its color. You should urinate within 1 hour of completing your run. Continue drinking fluids until the color of your urine is pale yellow.

Fueling After the Run

Whenever you run you deplete your glycogen stores, lose fluid and electrolytes, and damage muscle fibers. As soon as you complete your run, think recovery. Nutrition is as important immediately following your run as it was before and during your run. Quickly fueling your body after the run takes advantage of the body's ability to repair and restore to optimal levels. Fuel your body within 30 minutes of your run with a snack consisting of protein, carbohydrates, and fluids. Look for foods to provide at least 10 grams of protein. Protein aids in repair of damaged muscle tissue and stimulates development of new tissue. Consume 30–50 grams of carbohydrate to replenish depleted glycogen and also to enhance muscle repair. Examples of post-run fuel include smoothies with added protein, sports bars containing at least 10 grams of protein, chocolate milk, or a turkey sandwich.

QUESTION

What should I look for in an energy bar?
The energy bar you choose depends on its purpose. For before and during exercise, choose energy bars that provide mostly carbohydrates and are low in fiber and fat. For after exercise and for between-meal snacks, choose energy bars that contain at least a 1:3 ratio of protein to carbohydrates with less than 30 percent of the calories coming from fat.

Post-Run Scenario

I feel nauseous after my runs and can't eat anything for a few hours. What can I do to get in my post-run nutrition?

If you are feeling nauseous after your runs, think about what you are eating and drinking before and during your run. Before the run make sure you are consuming easily digestible foods low in fat and fiber.

During your run, experiment with other beverages and carbohydrate sources to see if others are better tolerated. When finished with your run, try drinking 4–8 ounces of a carbonated beverage such as ginger ale or even a cola to help settle your stomach. You'll accomplish ingesting carbs and fluid by consuming this beverage. If that works you can move on to consuming a healthier snack or meal for continued replenishment.

What Do "Real" Runners Eat?

Who do you look to for nutrition advice? Do you look to other runners? Below are two runners who did well in their sport.

Mary is a 40-year-old runner who has been running all of her adult life. She trains for one half-marathon a year and otherwise runs 5K and 10K races. Mary is 5'5" tall and weighs 130 pounds. Her best running times occurred when she was in her 30s. She often won her age group in local races.

Mary's typical daily diet consisted of:

- **Breakfast:** Coffee, 2 cups shredded wheat, 1 cup milk, 1 banana, ¼ cup walnuts
- **Midmorning snack:** A 200-calorie snack of yogurt and mixed fruit
- **Lunch:** Turkey and cheese sandwich with mayo, pretzels, apple, 2 medium cookies
- **Afternoon snack:** Almonds and pretzels
- **Dinner:** Chicken breast, baked potato with pat of butter, 1 cup broccoli, ear of corn, glass of wine
- **Before-bed snack:** 2 cookies and a glass of skim milk

The night before a race, Mary would do best on a small lean steak, big baked potato, green beans, and water. The common pre-race pasta dinner was just not for her.

Mary was a consistent eater and a consistent runner. Although a close evaluation might show areas of improvement in her diet, she ate a diet she enjoyed and was thoughtful in what worked for her (steak over pasta). She provided her body with nutrients and energy, and kept her weight consistent. Bravo!

John is a 35-year-old runner who ran weekly with Mary. John once won local races or placed in the top five when he was in his 20s. John lives on sports drinks, granola bars, jellybeans, and hamburgers. Here's John's typical daily intake:

- **Breakfast:** 2 granola bars and 16 ounces of sports drink
- **Midmorning:** Jellybeans and 16 ounces of sports drink
- **Lunch:** Burger and fries and 16 ounces of sports drinks
- **Afternoon snack:** 16 ounces of sports drink and a granola bar
- **Dinner:** Chicken sandwich and fries, iced tea
- **Before bed:** 16 ounces of sports drink

John had the genetic edge. And yet, as John got older, his weight crept up and his times got slower. Both his weight and his nutrition probably contributed to his slower performance. He is now working to eat smarter and is looking to Mary for advice.

"Real" runners eat in a variety of ways, sometimes following what research tells us is helpful and healthful and sometimes not. For the best likelihood of optimal performance and energy, however, follow the sports nutrition guidelines, not necessarily what fellow runners eat.

Popular Diets

Runners often look for the magic bullet to help them run faster, get leaner, and feel better. This makes diet books and supplements appealing. But do they work? Let's take a look at the evidence for a few popular diets.

The Paleolithic Diet

The Paleolithic Diet is often shortened as the Paleo diet. It is the diet plan that best resembles how early cavemen ate thousands of years ago, eating plants and wild animals. Meat, fish, shellfish, eggs, tree nuts, vegetables, roots, fruits, and berries are allowed, while grains and dairy are prohibited. A major advantage of this diet is that processed foods are eliminated and foods high in protein, vitamins, minerals, phytochemicals, and antioxidants are consumed.

The creators of the Paleo diet adapted it for athletes, recognizing that athletes do need more carbohydrates before, during, and after exercising. The Paleo diet for athletes allows for inclusion of grains and higher glycemic carbohydrates, especially for recovery after exercise.

If following a Paleo diet, one needs to consume enough variety to obtain all of the nutrients needed for optimal health. Following this diet by picking and choosing only certain foods can lead to deficiencies. Since it is toughest to consume enough calcium and vitamin D with this diet, it may be wise to take a calcium and vitamin D supplement. At this writing there is no conclusive evidence that this particular diet is superior to others in optimizing health and performance.

The Raw Food Diet

Raw foodism is a belief that plant foods in their most natural state are the most wholesome for the body. The raw food diet is 75 percent fruits and vegetables. Food choices include seaweed, sprouts, whole grains, beans, and nuts. Food preparation involves a food dehydrator that heats to a temperature no higher than 118 degrees Fahrenheit so that vitamins, minerals, and food enzymes are not destroyed.

Although many benefits can be achieved through a high fruit and vegetable diet, some fruits and vegetables are more available to the body when cooked. For example, the lycopene in tomatoes is more beneficial for the body when the tomatoes are cooked. Foods prepared at temperatures at or below 118 degrees may not destroy all harmful, food-borne bacteria and can be dangerous. People following this diet may have difficulty obtaining sufficient vitamin B12, calcium, iron, and omega-3 fatty acids, thus requiring supplementation.

Special Considerations for Female Athletes

Males and females are not built the same way. The ideal body compositions of a male and female body are quite different. Contrary to a male, whose body is 3–5 percent essential fat, the essential fat on a female body is 11–13 percent. Body fat serves a purpose—to cushion organs—and in females it prepares the body for reproduction. Although variable, most females require a minimum of 17 percent body fat for normal menstruation. And, although many women don't mind not having menstrual periods, the monthly cycle does more for a female than prepare it for reproduction. Among many functions, the hormones associated with a menstrual period, especially estrogen, are important for brain and bone growth and development. Females with low body fat and without menstrual periods (amenorrhea) are more likely to have stress fractures, premature osteoporosis, and an inability to conceive. The combination of low body weight (low body fat) and amenorrhea is a strong predictor of osteoporosis, regardless of the amount of weight-bearing exercise or calcium consumed in the diet.

The Female Athlete Triad

For some runners, more commonly women, running is not just a pleasurable activity that enhances fitness and reduces stress, it is a means to an end—to lose weight and especially to lose body fat. Although males and females alike seek to have a lean body, the female runner tends to have a greater obsession and drive toward thinness. Low caloric intake and high-energy expenditure from exercise—that is, energy-deficient, disordered eating; osteoporosis, or weakened bones; and amenorrhea result in what is referred to as the female athletic triad. Excess exercise without sufficient fuel results in compromised nutritional status, early fatigue, immune suppression, bone loss, stress fractures, and osteoporosis.

The body requires a certain number of calories just for vital bodily processes to occur. Approximately 70 percent of your calorie needs are used to fuel the vital organs (heart, lung, kidneys, liver, brain). You deprive your vital organs of needed energy when you eat only enough calories to make up for the calories you burned in exercise.

Some women and a growing number of men driven to thinness and body image struggle with disordered eating and even eating disorders that trap them into an obsession to undereat and overexercise. Although disordered eating is commonly believed to occur predominantly among women, the National Eating Disorders Association estimates that more than 1 million men and boys in the United States also struggle with eating disorders. If you find yourself in this unhealthy trap, seek help. Visit the NEDA website, *www.edap.org,* to learn more about eating disorders and find resources in your area to get the professional help you need.

Iron-Deficiency Anemia

Another issue that occurs more often with females than males is iron-deficiency anemia. When iron stores are low, fatigue increases and performance suffers. Iron is a component of hemoglobin, the protein in red blood cells that moves oxygen through the blood from the lungs to the working muscles. Without adequate oxygen moving to the working muscles, you cannot perform at your best, and you live in a state of fatigue. The recommended amount of iron to consume each day is 8 milligrams for men and 18 milligrams for menstruating women. Post-menopausal women should consume 8 milligrams of iron per day.

FACT

Signs of iron deficiency anemia include pale skin, shortness of breath, elevated heart rate, headaches, dizziness, loss of appetite, coldness in the hands and feet, and fatigue. You may also notice brittle nails and swelling of the tongue. Cravings for nonfood items such as ice, dirt, and starch occur in rare cases.

Women athletes are at a high risk for developing iron-deficiency anemia because of the loss of iron through monthly menstrual bleeding, along with the breakdown of red blood cells containing iron that occurs from the footstrike against the pavement while running. Endurance athletes may also lose iron through sweat. If you're feeling easily fatigued, it is a good idea to ask your health care professional to check your iron status, and in particular your ferritin levels. Ferritin, a protein that binds with iron, measures the iron stores in your body. Checking ferritin levels is not routine but can reveal a pre-anemia state.

Iron is best consumed through lean cuts of beef, pork, lamb, chicken, and turkey. The iron in animal foods is better absorbed into the body than plant sources of iron, such as dark green leafy vegetables like spinach. You can also obtain iron in enriched and fortified breads and cereals. Using a cast-iron skillet for cooking allows the food to absorb the iron for an enhanced benefit. Coffee and tea inhibit the absorption of iron and are best consumed an hour before or after a meal.

CHAPTER 5

Time to Get Going!

You're motivated, you're conscientious, you're equipped, and you have learned about proper mechanics. So, are you ready to go running? Or are you wondering where you should begin? If this is your first time running, read on to learn how to run and to review some important tips.

Starting Out

Even if you've never run a step in your life, the training schedule in Table 5-1 will enable you to become a runner in a matter of a few short weeks. Where you choose to begin this schedule depends on your current fitness level. If you're just getting into a cardiovascular exercise program, start at the beginning of Week 1 with brisk walking and proceed through the schedule as indicated. For individuals who currently are quite active (who, at a minimum, can easily walk at a brisk pace and/or jog nonstop for 2 minutes), begin following the schedule at Week 7.

To minimize your chance of incurring an injury, be patient and stick to the schedule. By all means, avoid the urge to do more than is specified. During the early weeks of the schedule, feel free to break up the cumulative minutes indicated for running into smaller segments if you feel it necessary. There's no problem in modifying the schedule to fit into your busy lifestyle so long as you keep the sequence of runs the same. For example, if Sunday is not a good day for you to run, the time and/or mileage goal indicated on that day can be shifted to another day of the week so long as the sequence for the remainder of runs during the week is also shifted.

The pace of your running should be at an aerobic level (meaning the ability to breathe easily without pushing yourself). In other words, you should be running very relaxed and comfortably. You should be able to talk in complete sentences without gasping for air. In the beginning the key to success and evaluation of your progress should be based on the *cumulative minutes* you are able to run without stopping rather than on the pace at which you run. With consistent training over a period of weeks, your running form will become more refined and efficient. This in itself often translates into a faster pace without the need to overload your present musculoskeletal system.

The purpose of light weeks (also referred to as *step-back weeks* by some coaches) is to facilitate rest and recovery from systematic increases in time and distance the previous weeks. Contrary to what you might think, light weeks enable you to gather strength for the next progression upward.

▼ **TABLE 5-1: BEGINNER RUN/WALK SCHEDULE**

Week #	Sun.	Mon.	Tue.	Wed.	Thur.	Fri.	Sat.	Total
1	W-8	Rest	W-10	Rest	W-11	Rest	W-8	W-37
2	W-12	Rest	W-14	Rest	W-16	Rest	W-10	W-52
3	W-18	Rest	W-20	Rest	W-22	Rest	W-12	W-72
4	W-24	Rest	W-26	Rest	W-28	Rest	W-12	W-90
5	W-30	Rest	W-30	Rest	W-30	Rest	W-30	W-120
6	W-20	Rest	W-20	Rest	W-26	Rest	W-20	W-86 Light Week
7	R-2 W-28	Rest	R-3 W-27	Rest	R-4 W-26	Rest	W-30	R-9 W-131
8	R-5 W-25	Rest	R-6 W-24	Rest	R-8 W-22	Rest	R-6 W-24	R-25 W-95
9	R-10 W-20	Rest	R-11 W-19	Rest	R-12 W-18	Rest	R-8 W-22	R-41 W-79
10	R-14 W-16	Rest	R-16 W-14	Rest	R-18 W-12	Rest	R-10 W-20	R-58 W-62
11	R-20 W-10	Rest	R-22 W-8	Rest	R-24 W-6	Rest	R-12 W-18	R-78 W-42
12	R-26 W-4	Rest	R-28 W-2	Rest	R-30	Rest	R-14 W-16	R-98 W-22
13	R-20	Rest	R-20 W-10	Rest	R-26 W-4	Rest	R-16 W-14	R-82 W-28 Light Week
14	R-30	Rest	R-25 W-5	Rest	R-30	Rest	R-18 W-12	R-103 W-17
15	R-33	Rest	R-30	Rest	R-30	Rest	R-20 W-10	R-113 W-10
16	R-36	Rest	R-30	Rest	R-30	Rest	R-20 W-10	R-116 W-10
17	R-39	Rest	R-30	Rest	R-30	Rest	R-30	R-129
18	R-20 W-10	Rest	R-20 W-10	Rest	R-26 W-4	Rest	R-20 W-10	R-86 W-34 Light Week

W = Walk; R = Run; Numbers = Minutes of exercise

Even if your goal is to run, don't ever be ashamed to walk. In fact, the first sections of the beginner schedule feature a mixture of walking and running. If you are unable to run the specified time and/or mileage goal on the schedule at the present time, then by all means walk the distance.

Learning How to Run

Even if you haven't exercised in years, if you can walk for 15 or 20 minutes, this schedule can make you a runner. It can also take you to your first 5K in eighteen weeks!

When starting out, have fun, and don't give in to the desire to do too much too soon—or worse, don't quit before you reap the benefits that running can provide. Be patient with yourself and consistent in your workout. In short, enjoy the process, but don't overdo it. Happiness in running comes from the journey, not with the final destination.

Tips Before You Begin

Before you head out the door, review the following tips. Even though running is a simple activity, you need to be mindful of what you're doing at all times in order to maximize its benefits and your enjoyment.

- Be aware of road and trail slants
- Stay hydrated
- Mind the seasons
- Minimize risks
- Let others help

Runners should pay attention to road or trail slants and camber (the slightly arched shape of the road or trail surface), regardless of whether they have hip or knee problems. Frequent running on pitched or slanted surfaces increases your chances of incurring injury. If your knees or hips are prone to soreness, you should pay special attention to the camber and try to run on the flattest, most level portion. This will reduce the angular stress that can make any injury a more serious problem.

FACT

The shortest distance between two points is a straight line. In training, it is fine to hug the wide lines, such as running along the outside edges of course curves, for example. But when you are running in a road race or timed event, look for and run the shortest official course, especially on curves and turns. Hugging the outside border of the road can add mileage and time to your performance.

For hot, humid days and for runs of more than half an hour, it is very important that you drink fluids every 25–30 minutes. Above all, don't wait until you're thirsty to start taking in fluids. Before setting out, drink 8 ounces of water and hydrate regularly during your run. Be careful, though, not to drink excessive amounts of water as doing so can lead to the dangerous condition of hyponatremia. For runs lasting an hour or longer, it is important to also consume sports drinks such as Gatorade® or Powerade®. You can also plan your route so that you are able to stop at water fountains along the way. Doing so offers the psychological advantage of breaking up the run mentally, since you can set yourself the goal of running from one fluid stop to the next.

Certainly one of the great things about running is that it is a year-round sport. You can run through every season as long as you adequately hydrate and dress appropriately. Dress warmly enough in winter and dress to stay cool enough in summer. Be especially careful on extremely hot or cold days. You should always try to avoid running in extreme heat and extreme cold. If you really must run in such conditions, bring plenty of fluids with you and consider shortening your workout for that day.

Cautions

Running, like many other sports, poses its own set of potential problems, including dangers on the trail and risk of injury. One of the most important things you can do is to be aware of your surroundings. Keep your head up and your eyes focused ahead of you rather than down at your feet. If you run in the dark, make yourself visible to others by way of reflective clothing, decals, or tape. Carry a small flashlight so you can see where you are landing.

Let someone know where you are going, what time you are leaving, and when you expect to return. No matter what distance you plan to run, consider carrying your cell phone so you won't be stranded if you incur injury or need help of any type. At the same time, a word to the wise: Don't consider your running time a chance to catch up on phone calls. Even though carrying a cell phone is a smart safety feature, resist the temptation to use it unless you have a real emergency.

On a dirt trail, watch out for roots and rocks. Avoid running alone in areas that bears and mountain lions call home. For safety reasons, women should find companions to accompany them when running in unpopulated areas. Dogs and human companions can be fun accompaniments to running, and they provide security against undesired interactions.

FACT

Different degrees of pain after a workout can include soreness (a light achy feeling), aches (continuous dull throbbing), and pains (acute and sharp hurting). If soreness or aches don't diminish, take some time off from running. If pain increases, stay off the injury, apply RICE (rest, ice, compress, elevation), and take a pain reliever. If the pain doesn't subside in a few days, see a doctor.

Don't overdo it, especially in the beginning. One of the negative effects of running excessive mileage or running too frequently (that is, not scheduling regular rest days) is the risk of incurring injury. Injuries to the knees, hips, and Achilles tendons, in particular, can often be attributed to overtraining. Listen to your body, and don't make comparisons between your training program and the mileage totals of other runners.

Stay Motivated

Making this change in your life by taking up running is a big deal and something you should feel really good about. Make a copy of whichever training schedule you choose from this book and put it in a prominent place in your home. With the schedule clearly displayed, you can chart your progress. In fact, you can keep yourself motivated by asking your housemates to help you stay on track. That way, when you meet your goals, they can share in your success and help celebrate what has become truly a group effort. This might even inspire someone you live with to join you in running.

Stretching Fundamentals

Before you get started on any serious running program, you'll need to learn how to stretch. Stretching properly is one of the most important steps you can take to lessen your chances of injury, whether you're a beginner or a veteran marathoner. Whenever you stretch, remember the objectives of stretching, which are to improve flexibility and lengthen your muscles so they can perform optimally, and to reduce your chances of suffering from an injury. When you integrate stretching into your overall workout routine, you'll be amazed by how much better you'll feel all over.

How to Stretch Properly

Have you ever seen someone go about stretching haphazardly? He throws his foot onto a fence post or railing, awkwardly bends toward it, bounces a few times, tries to grab his foot a couple of times, then heaves his foot back down and starts with the other one. Your common sense should tell you that there's something wrong with this all-too-common sight, and indeed there is.

To be effective, stretching needs to be slow, gentle, and focused. Concentrate on the muscles or muscle groups you're working on and breathe naturally and regularly (no holding your breath). Inhale as you set up the stretch, then exhale as you lean into the stretch, moving slowly to gently extend the muscle to its full length. Stop when you feel mild tension and hold the stretch for 30–60 seconds. At the end of that time, inhale out of the stretch as gently as you went into it.

Patience Is a Virtue

Even if you begin with poor flexibility, a regular stretching program will greatly improve your range of motion. The key is to be both patient and consistent. Your stretching should not cause pain, although it may feel a bit uncomfortable at first or even awkward when you begin a stretching regimen.

You can supplement your stretching with exercises to improve your posture and physical strength. Core strengthening and exercises to improve your upper- and lower-body strength can benefit your overall health and improve your running.

Static stretch basics include:

- Stretch the muscle to the point of its greatest length, but don't overstretch.
- Never bounce when stretching; instead, hold the stretch for 30–60 seconds.
- Stretch the major leg muscle groups.
- Stretch uniformly (after stretching one leg, stretch the other).
- Don't overstretch an injured area, as this may cause additional damage.

The Best Stretches for Runners

The stretches described here benefit the major muscles in your legs—those that control your ankles, knees, and hips.

Stretching the Calves

Having tight calves is a strong predictor for injuries such as Achilles tendinitis, plantar fasciitis, and calf strain. A common calf stretch performed by runners is done by standing with one foot in front of the other and your hands on a wall or tree. Point both feet straight ahead and gently lean forward, keeping the heel of your back foot on the ground and your knee straight. Perform two 20-second holds in this position (stretching the calf of the back leg); then shift your weight back, bend your knee slightly, and perform two more 20-second stretches on this same leg. Next, switch legs and repeat the stretches on the other leg.

Stretching the Hamstrings

Tight hamstrings can lead to muscle strain and even lower back pain. To stretch hamstring muscles out, stand with your feet shoulder-width apart and pointing straight ahead. Bend over at the waist, reaching your hands toward your feet. Keep your knees slightly bent as you do this and only go as far down as it takes to feel a gentle stretch.

As you bend down, relax your neck and shoulders, and slowly exhale. When you reach the slightly tight point, relax into it and hold for approximately 30 seconds. Then start straightening back up as you inhale. Move slowly, and allow your head to roll up gently as well. When you're back in the standing position, exhale. Inhale as you begin to bend forward again.

Repeat this stretch three to five times. If you do this after every run, you'll notice improvements in your flexibility within a week. Soon you'll be able to reach your knees, then your ankles, and—yes—your toes!

Another way to stretch your hamstrings is by performing an *active* hamstring stretch, one called "Bottoms Up." Squat with your knees bent, your back relaxed, and your forearms resting on your thighs. Straighten your knees by contracting your thigh muscles while keeping your forearms on your thighs. Feel the stretch in your hamstrings and hold for 10 seconds. Repeat three to five times.

There are a number of ways to stretch your hamstrings; most of them are passive stretches. Clinical evidence suggests that the active hamstring stretching, such as the "Bottoms Up" stretch, is most effective for lengthening muscle.

Stretching the Quadriceps

Your *quadricep* muscles are located on the front of your thighs. One way to stretch them is done in the standing position. To stretch your right quad, support yourself with your right hand on a wall or railing. Bend your right knee while grabbing your foot behind you with your left hand. With your toes slightly pointed, gently bring your foot toward your buttocks as you exhale. Hold the stretch for about 30 seconds. Switch legs. Repeat until you've stretched both legs two to three times. You can also work on improving your balance with this stretch by steadying yourself on the leg you're standing on and removing your hand from the wall or railing.

The *quadriceps muscles* (quads) and *iliotibial band* (IT band) control the knee during exercise. The quads are the four muscles in the front of your thigh; the IT band runs from your hip to your knee along the outside of your leg.

The "Lower Body All-Over" Stretch

This stretch, sometimes called the squat stretch, is a great stretch for your lower back, ankles, Achilles tendons, shins, and groin. If you spend a lot of time sitting or standing, you'll come to love this stretch. However, if you're a beginner, it can be particularly tough—go easy!

Stand with your feet shoulder-width apart and your toes pointing out slightly. Keeping your feet flat, slowly lower yourself into a squat. Exhale. Your knees should be outside of your shoulders but over your big toes. Support yourself with your arms in front of you and between your legs, hands touching the floor (if possible). You may want to do this with your back against a wall for additional support.

When you're squatting, hold the stretch for about 30 seconds. Come up slowly, inhaling as you straighten. Repeat two to three times when you're first learning this stretch. As you get better, hold it for a bit longer, and see if you can repeat it four to five times.

Stretching the Piriformis Muscle

The *piriformis* muscle extends from the hip to the sacrum (the bone at the base of the spine that attaches to the pelvis). The piriformis stretch can help keep you flexible through the hips. There are several ways to stretch the piriformis. One method is performed by sitting on the ground with one leg straight and the other bent at the knee. Use both hands to take the foot and knee of the bent leg and pull them toward your chest. You will feel the stretch in the buttock area of the leg you are cradling toward your chest. Hold for about 30 seconds, and switch legs. Repeat two to three times with each leg.

Working with a Professional

Whether you are a beginner or an experienced competitive runner, there are many reasons to consider a personal training service. These include:

- To properly begin a running program from square one
- To train to complete short events, from the 5K to half-marathon
- To complete your first marathon safely and successfully
- To improve upon your finish time and conditioning level from a previous race
- To give structure to your training in the face of a busy lifestyle
- To provide an accountability component by reporting your progress, making it more likely that you'll stick to your training plan
- To maximize the benefits of training while reducing the chances of injury
- To take your running to the next level

When considering a personal coach, think about what you want from a coach and understand what you can and can't expect. Typical components of a personal training program include:

- Telephone consultations on a weekly basis
- E-mail support
- Goal-setting assistance
- Individualized training program based on your goals and needs
- Analysis of progress with adjustments based on your results
- Injury prevention guidance
- Nutritional tips
- Answers to your training questions
- Ongoing motivation and support

If you decide to opt for the services of a personal coach, research coaches in your area by talking to other runners, whom you can find through local running clubs.

Beginning Your Running Program

Remember that the safest and most enjoyable approach to running is to build up your ability incrementally. By following the suggestions and schedules in this book, you will find that your ability as a runner increases safely and steadily.

FACT

> "I've been running since I was in my thirties, and had never broken the barrier from a few minutes to long distance. Until Art Liberman put me on a training program—and it worked. Beginning with 12 minutes, I am now able to run 90-plus minutes nonstop."—Margo Painter, Pensacola, FL

Building a Base

Without question, the most important area one should focus on prior to beginning any running program is safely and slowly building your mileage. In anticipation of entering races longer than 10K (6.2 miles), you should eventually be running four to five days a week with minimum weekly mileage totals of 20–25 miles. At that point, longer runs and weekly mileage can be added in small increments. You should not introduce advanced running techniques, such as speed work and hill repeats, into your training schedule until you're physically ready.

Going to the Next Level

Assuming you have either completed the walk/run schedule or can run 4 miles prior to picking up this book, you can use the mileage buildup schedules in Tables 5-2 and 5-3 to prepare to run a 10-mile race. If you already have some running experience and wish to enter races longer than 10 miles, such as the half-marathon (13.1 miles) and marathon, in the near future, put your current training on hold until you systematically progress though the last couple of weeks of these schedules.

Prior to your target race, include a tapering-off period of 1–2 weeks in which you reduce your mileage totals 35–40 percent. By doing so, you will be well rested and ready to perform optimally come race day. For true beginners, use the walk/run schedule in Table 5-2 to set the stage for completing your first 5K (rather than for the goal of running it competitively).

The 10 Percent Rule

Do not increase either your weekly mileage or your long-run mileage by more than 10 percent a week. Doing so greatly increases the chances of incurring an injury, thereby delaying or stopping your training altogether. Many running injuries can be attributed to runners not following this simple but extremely important premise.

▼ TABLE 5-2: MILEAGE BUILDUP SCHEDULE

Week #	Sun.	Mon.	Tue.	Wed.	Thur.	Fri.	Sat.	Total
1	4	Rest	3	Rest	4	Rest	3	14
2	4	Rest	4	Rest	4	Rest	3	15
3	5	Rest	4	Rest	4	Rest	3	16
4	3	Rest	3	Rest	3	Rest	3	12 Light Week
5	5	Rest	4	Rest	4	Rest	4	17
6	6	Rest	4	Rest	4	Rest	4	18
7	6	Rest	4	Rest	5	Rest	4	19
8	3	Rest	4	Rest	3	Rest	3	13 Light Week
9	7	Rest	4	Rest	5	Rest	4	20
10	7	Rest	5	Rest	5	Rest	4	21
11	8	Rest	5	Rest	5	Rest	4	22
12	4	Rest	3	Rest	4	Rest	4	15 Light Week
13	8	Rest	5	Rest	6	Rest	4	23
14	9	Rest	5	Rest	6	Rest	4	24
15	9	Rest	6	Rest	6	Rest	4	25
16	5	Rest	4	Rest	4	Rest	4	17 Light Week
17	10	Rest	6	Rest	6	Rest	4	26
18	10	Rest	6	Rest	7	Rest	4	27
19	6	Rest	4	Rest	5	Rest	4	19 Light Week

Numbers (except week numbers) refer to miles of running

▼ **TABLE 5-3: ADVANCED MILEAGE BUILDUP SCHEDULE**

Week #	Sun.	Mon.	Tue.	Wed.	Thur.	Fri.	Sat.	Total
1	4	Rest	3	Rest	4	Rest	3	14
2	4	Rest	4	Rest	4	Rest	3	15
3	5	Rest	4	Rest	4	Rest	3	16
4	3	Rest	3	Rest	3	Rest	3	12 Light Week
5	5	Rest	3	3	3	Rest	3	17
6	6	Rest	3	3	3	Rest	3	18
7	6	Rest	3	4	3	Rest	4	20
8	3	Rest	4	Rest	3	Rest	3	13 Light Week
9	7	Rest	3	5	4	Rest	3	22
10	7	Rest	4	5	4	Rest	4	24
11	8	Rest	4	6	4	Rest	4	26
12	4	Rest	3	Rest	4	Rest	4	15 Light Week
13	8	Rest	5	6	5	Rest	4	28
14	9	Rest	5	5	6	Rest	4	29
15	9	Rest	5	7	6	Rest	5	32
16	5	Rest	4	Rest	4	Rest	4	17 Light Week
17	10	Rest	6	8	6	Rest	4	34
18	10	Rest	6	8	7	Rest	4	35
19	6	Rest	4	Rest	5	Rest	4	19 Light Week

Numbers refer to miles of running

Beginning Runner's Mistakes

Watch out for common mistakes that beginning runners often make. These include:

- **Focusing on speed.** Try to focus on increasing your duration rather than your speed as a means of evaluating your progress.
- **Doing too much too soon.** Increasing mileage as a result of overenthusiasm often leads to the most common beginner running injury—Medial Tibial Stress Syndrome (MTSS) (formerly called "shin splints").

- **Not listening to your body.** If excessively sore or fatigued, either walk or take an extra day off. Don't be a slave to your training schedule!
- **Using old running shoes, shoes not designed specifically for running, or shoes that are not appropriate for your biomechanical needs.**
- **Training with the wrong people.** Run with others who share your level of ability, not with those who run either much faster or much slower than you.
- **Trying to emulate other people's running styles.** Use the proper form when you run to avoid discomfort or injury.
- **Giving up too soon.** If you find yourself getting discouraged soon after you start a running program, be careful not to talk yourself out of it. Re-evaluate the reasons you wanted to start running. Ask yourself what happened between having those feelings and becoming discouraged. Are your expectations unrealistic? Is there something about the process that doesn't feel right? Do you recognize any mistakes listed here as contributing to your feeling discouraged?

A More Advanced Schedule

When you complete your choice of buildup schedule, you will have developed a base from which you can now train for race distances longer than 10 miles. The advanced mileage buildup schedule features five days of training (on most weeks) and more weekly mileage than the previous mileage buildup schedule.

So how do you decide which schedule to choose? Some readers of this book are already at or above the level of the basic buildup schedule and will want other mileage buildup options. These runners have the time and desire to train five days a week. If this describes you, make sure you are up to it and can comfortably train at this level. Don't push yourself too hard by selecting a schedule that does not yet match your present level of conditioning.

At the conclusion of Week 19 of either schedule, assuming that you've made it through the mileage buildup stage without injury, you are now ready to proceed to new training goals. These might include incorporating more advanced training techniques (such as speed work) and/or training for longer races such as the half-marathon and marathon.

CHAPTER 6

The Mechanics of Running

Is there really a right way to run? Conversely, is there a wrong way to run? The answer to both questions is yes. However, that does not mean that everyone should run in the same way with the same form. The fact is that form varies from runner to runner. Every person's form emerges naturally over time. The objective of this chapter is to teach you about the fundamentals of form so you can maximize your natural running efficiencies and minimize the technique mistakes that can lead to injury.

Running Form Mistakes

Many of the fastest runners are not necessarily naturally gifted, nor are they necessarily tall or long-limbed. Instead, the best runners are those with economical strides who run with purpose, power, and determination. Not only can good form make the difference between running pain-free and running with pain, but if you are a racer, good form can also shave minutes off your running time.

Improving one's speed poses the greatest challenge for a runner. Many runners, both beginners and intermediates, lean too far forward and run on their toes in an attempt to run faster. Running on your toes, or forefoot, is a sprinting technique only. If you try running a 5K or 10K race like this, you will probably end up in pain and maybe even injured.

Speed and efficiency can also be negatively affected by bouncing. Bouncing up and down while you run slows you down and is extremely inefficient. Bouncers tend to lope and overstride, which creates greater impact on your legs, especially on your knees.

There is a variety of other subtle form flaws that plague runners. Many of these problems are not readily recognizable. However, once identified, many flaws in technique can be easily corrected. Although you don't need to have perfect form, even a minor adjustment or modification can make a tremendous difference in your running efficiency and comfort level. Additionally, tweaking your form a bit can reduce your chances of incurring an injury.

Style and Mechanics

Your running style refers to the form and technique of how you run. Beginning runners should try running as naturally as possible while keeping in mind the proper biomechanics (explained below). Learning these mechanics leads to more efficient form. Don't push yourself to run fast right away. Instead, concentrate first on comfort and form. If you are new to the sport, it is best to approach running as a new lifestyle. To adopt this lifestyle you must first learn the correct habits and then perfect them. After you've been running for a few months, ask an experienced runner or (preferably) a coach to critique your form and point out any flaws or deficiencies. This can improve your overall mechanics and running efficiency.

PRINCIPLES TO KEEP IN MIND WHEN YOU RUN:

- **Run relaxed.** Keep your jaw and wrists relaxed as you run. The tension of holding your muscles tight saps energy and causes early fatigue.
- **Run naturally.** Develop your own running style while employing good running mechanics.
- **Run tall.** Activate your core to maintain good posture while you run. This will generate other good habits like optimal knee lift, natural extension of stride, and improved breathing.

Biomechanics are the individual components of movement that occur in the body during running. These components of movement include: breathing, footstrike, stride, arm swing, and posture. Each of these areas can affect your efficiency, your comfort, and your form.

Although you cannot change your body type or your bone and muscle structure, you can become a smoother, more efficient runner by correcting bad habits you may have unknowingly developed. By knowing the basics of good biomechanics, you can improve your running form.

Breathing

One of the most vital yet underrated areas that you can work on to improve your running efficiency is to correct a faulty breathing technique. The problem is that many people breathe from their chest rather than from their abdominal region while they run. Abdominal, or belly breathing, is the best method to inhale air deep into your lungs where most of the gas exchange between oxygen and carbon monoxide occurs.

FACT

A secret to breathing better when you run is to remember to put a little more force into your exhalation. Your body will naturally inhale to make up for this, which in turn will improve your breathing efficiency.

Whether you're a beginner or an experienced runner, take the time to learn and employ the abdominal breathing method. As a minimum, just remember to keep breathing deeply and regularly. In most cases your breathing will take care of itself; as you run faster, you'll breathe faster. And yes, most runners are mouth-breathers or at least nose-and-mouth breathers. It would be impossible to take in adequate oxygen by breathing only through your nose.

Your breathing shouldn't be labored. If you find yourself huffing and puffing, you are probably running too fast for your current level of fitness. Run at a pace where you can speak comfortably in complete sentences. In other words, your pace should be such that you're not gasping for air after each couple of words.

Establishing Your Breathing Rhythm

Your breathing rhythm is an important component of efficient and complete gas exchange in your lungs. Rhythm and stride are closely related to your breathing, so it is natural to learn to synchronize your stride with your breathing as you learn proper biomechanics. Whether you take three strides for every breath or two, your breathing and your stride are probably in sync naturally. Beginning runners, though, make the mistake of breathing at a 1:1 rate. This means that they are taking one step while breathing in and the next step while breathing out. This essentially is panting, and it is inefficient breathing.

A more economical way to breathe depends, to a large degree, on the pace at which you are running. For your average run, you should breathe 2:2—taking two steps for every breath in and two steps for every breath out—or 3:3 for longer, slower runs. As you run faster, you may have to breathe more often, which leads to such variations as 2:1 and 1:2 patterns.

All about Footstrike

Footstrike is the position that your foot first strikes the ground as you run. A footprint is the mark on the ground that you leave behind. Each footprint is like your signature as a runner. Do you run on your toes? Do you run heel to toe? Do you run flat-footed? The way your foot makes contact with the ground is very important. If your foot does not properly control your landing, then some corrections need to be made. These corrections may include being fitted for the proper shoes to match the biomechanical needs of your foot or maybe adding an orthotic or arch support to your shoes.

FACT

Short- and middle-distance runners naturally first strike the ground with their forefoot or midfoot. Long-distance and beginning runners wearing heavy, cushioned, high-heeled running shoes develop a heel-strike form. Experts in the field are examining whether heel striking for long-distance runners should be replaced by midfoot striking. At this writing, there is no evidence to support the premise that heel-striking leads to fewer injuries; in fact, just the opposite may be true.

Mechanics of the Foot

There are three basic types of footstrikes: normal/neutral, overpronated, and supinated (also called underpronated). In the normal, or neutral, footstrike, the foot rolls slightly inward as it strikes. Your foot flattens out as it makes full contact with the ground, then rolls inward as your body passes over your foot. This inward roll of your foot while running, called pronation, is actually a good thing, since it absorbs some of the force placed on the leg during normal running. Following normal pronation, your foot will naturally resupinate (roll outward) to allow the foot to form a rigid lever for push-off.

Only about 25 percent of the population pronates normally, however, leaving the rest to figure out how to compensate. Overpronation occurs when the foot rolls inward excessively and does not resupinate in time for push-off. When the foot is overpronated, the push-off occurs from the big toe and not evenly across the toes as it should. Overpronation is oftentimes seen in those who have flat feet or in those with poor motor control of their feet while running. Running shoe models designed and constructed with motion control or stability features help reduce the degree of overpronation. This in turn helps prevent a wide array of overuse injuries that can occur if overpronation is left unchecked.

Supination, or underpronation, also occurs when the outside of the heel makes initial contact with the ground. The foot of the supinator fails to roll inward enough as the body passes over the foot, resulting in the outside of the foot taking too much of the load, and push-off being done by the smaller toes. Characteristic of runners with high, rigid arches, supination minimizes the ability of the foot—and, in turn, the legs—to absorb shock, which can lead to injury. To counteract supination, runners with this type of footstrike should wear running shoes that are well-cushioned and flexible. It's important to know whether you are a normal pronator, an overpronator, or a supinator *before* you buy your running shoes so that you can get a pair that helps compensate appropriately.

Some experts believe that the issue of excessive pronation or supination can be minimized or eliminated altogether by incorporating a midfoot strike pattern. This belief is what fuels the barefoot and minimalist shoes running movement. Studies are ongoing.

QUESTION

Which foot type are you?
Give yourself a footprint test to determine this. While barefoot, put a piece of cardboard on the floor, wet the bottom of your foot, and press firmly with a solid walking motion on the cardboard to leave an impression of the bottom of your foot in motion. If your footprint appears flat and shows almost your entire foot, you are probably an overpronator. If your footprint shows little or no connecting band between your heel and the ball of your foot, you probably have high arches and may be a supinator (underpronator).

The Toes' Role in Footstrike

Regardless of what kind of footstrike you have, you need to keep in mind your toes. Sometimes, especially when you are tired, your feet don't always point forward when you run. If it is not totally awkward for you, try to run with your toes pointed forward. Doing so will result in greater efficiency, which in turn enables you to run faster and farther with the same cardiovascular effort. Running with your foot turned out will cause you to push off with your big toe, which is poor biomechanically and puts excessive stress on your big toe and forefoot. In short, toes and feet that aren't pointed in the right direction result in wasted and inefficient motion and can result in injury.

Of course, this advice is intended for those who need to adjust faulty technique in order to improve their form to reduce their chances of injury. Some runners are not built in such a way that allows them to have a "perfect" footfall. For them, a forced effort to run a certain way can actually create a problem worse than poor running form.

ESSENTIAL

Go for a run paying particular attention to your footstrike. Have a friend videotape you running. Watching yourself run allows you to see your running style and may show some obvious form flaws that you can correct, which will make you a more efficient runner.

Flat, Heel, and Toe Footstrikes

Many beginners run with a *flat* footstrike, characterized by landing on a flat foot and having little or no push-off. This isn't particularly bad or wrong. If this is the way you run, especially in the beginning, don't change it. Run naturally. To improve your speed and overall efficiency, however, you will eventually need to make some adjustments to your footstrike and push-off.

The *heel-strike* pattern is the most common footstrike of runners (approximately 80 percent of all runners heel-strike). With a heel-strike, at the initial contact with the ground your heel lands first, then you roll along the outer border of your foot until your midfoot makes contact with the ground. Finally, your toes make contact with the ground as your heel lifts up, and your foot lifts off the ground. If this is how you run, you may or may not want to change this, at least not when you first begin a running program. It is a very normal and natural footstrike that most runners who wear the modern high-heeled running shoes will adopt.

The heel-strike technique is perfectly fine for longer, slower running. However, as with the flat footstrike, to gain the speed and efficiency that shorter runs and races require, you should adopt the midfoot strike footprint.

Many beginners slap their feet on the ground when they run, creating too hard a footfall. Your foot should land *gently* on the ground if you are a heel-striker. If your feet are slapping the ground and making an audible noise when you run, you need to make a serious change. Land gently on each foot and lift each foot gently off the ground.

Another type of footstrike pattern is the *toe-strike*. This is a footstrike in which only your toes and forefoot make initial contact with the ground. This is a sprinting technique and is not appropriate for distance running. Therefore, unless you are a sprinter, don't purposely run on your toes.

FACT

In an attempt to improve their speed, many beginning runners compensate by employing either the heel or toe footstrike method. Over time, both methods increase the wear and tear on one's legs, so you may be best off running with a midfoot strike.

Heel-Ball and Ball-Heel-Toe Footstrikes

The method of footstrike most commonly adopted by the beginner, intermediate, and heavier runner is the *heel-ball strike*. (For the purpose of this discussion, the ball of your foot is the area that starts behind the base of your big toe and goes across the bottom of your foot to your smallest toe.) Although in the heel-ball footstrike the heel strikes first, the ball of the foot quickly follows. This footstrike allows for impact to be absorbed first by the cushioned heel of the shoe, then by your foot and leg.

A better footstrike technique is the ball-heel-toe strike, better known as the midfoot strike. When you midfoot-strike, you land on the outside edge of the midfoot, bring your foot down so your heel touches the ground, and then roll back up to push off with your big toe. This technique is used more often by advanced runners than by beginners. Because beginners are still in the process of developing strength in their feet and calves, they may develop muscle soreness and possibly increase their risk of injury by employing this footstrike style. The midfoot strike is appropriate to use when you can average less than 7 minutes per mile running pace.

It's All about Stride

The swing of your legs into position as you run is called your stride. Some people have long, loping strides, while others have short, economical ones. Some lift their knees high, while others barely lift them at all. Your stride can make a huge difference in how efficiently you run. Runners who want to increase their speed turn to adjusting their stride in order to advance to the next level.

Start with your natural stride, and see where it takes you. Don't be concerned with trying to run fast when you begin a running program. But as beginning runners progress through the first few months of their running program and want to improve their efficiency and speed, there are three adjustments that can be considered: stride frequency, stride length, and knee lift.

ALERT

Even though it has always been considered a good thing to have a little bounce in your step, in running circles it is a sign that something is wrong. Don't bounce or bound; it means that you are overstriding. If you shorten your stride and eliminate bouncing, you redirect energy that can be better used to propel yourself forward.

Stride Length

Stride length refers to how far you are stepping out when you extend your leg and foot. Increasing your stride length increases the amount of ground you cover with each step. However, make sure not to overextend your stride, since overstriding is inefficient.

A good rule of thumb is for your foot to strike the ground beneath your knee. Some running experts feel that a short stride is a sign of inflexibility. That is not always so. Proper stretching after a run can help to improve your flexibility, which can in turn lengthen your stride.

Overstriders are easy to spot because they tend to lope or bounce, and their motion is not rhythmic or fluid. Overstriding occurs when your foot lands in front of your center of gravity. When this happens, it causes a braking force that can actually slow you down.

Your optimal stride length occurs when your foot lands directly beneath your knee. This might feel like too short a stride at first, but a shorter stride is more efficient than a longer one.

ALERT

Don't kick your legs up when you run. Some runners kick their heels way up behind them when they run, wasting motion and energy. To get the optimum benefit from your stride, you should extend your leg behind you when pushing off, and then bring it forward as soon as possible.

Stride Frequency

Increasing the frequency of your stride is a little more challenging than increasing your stride length. Your stride frequency, also called "turnover," is defined as the number of steps you take in 1 minute. A shorter stride *length* will yield a higher stride *frequency*, whereas a long, loping stride leads to a slower turnover. A frequency of 140–180 steps per minute is ideal for distance running. For running techniques such as barefoot running or ChiRunning®, stride frequency of 170–180 steps per minute is preferred. One way to improve your stride frequency is by using a metronome when you run.

Knee Lift

By focusing on your knee motion, you'll probably improve both your stride frequency and stride length. Be careful not to bring your knees up too high, because how far up you bring your knees determines how long your stride will be. Remember, a stride that's too long or too short is inefficient. Therefore, the correct knee lift coupled with the correct frequency of leg turnover dictates how effectively you can cover ground. In short, the knees do not have to come up very high for long-distance runners. Only sprinters or those charging up a hill have to lift their legs a bit higher than usual.

Arms and Hands

Your arms help to provide balance and power while running. Many feel there is a correlation between moving their arms faster and getting their legs to move faster. Optimally, the arms should support the energy of the body in a forward motion while running.

Your arms provide balance in the following way: As your left leg goes forward, so does your right arm. This balances you as you move forward. Then when the right leg moves forward, so does the left arm. The way you carry your arms while moving is called "arm carriage."

For proper arm carriage, your hands should be lightly clasped (as though you are holding a roll of dimes) rather than tightly clinched. Don't waste muscle power needlessly. This isn't a stress test, so relax. Allow your arms to swing from the shoulder, with your wrists at the level of the waistband of your shorts. Make sure your hands are not too high or too low. Your elbows and wrists should be relaxed and not carrying any tension.

Different types of runners have different types of arm carriage. Sprinters pump their arms in a straight forward-backward motion. Most longer-distance runners use a slight arc as they swing their arms, but the faster, more efficient ones don't waste motion by moving too much from side to side. Remember, you want all motions of your body to be moving in the forward direction. This includes the motion of your arms in front of your body.

Wasted motion in the arms is just as bad as an improper or inefficient stride in the legs. A few arm carriage "Don'ts" include:

- Don't carry your arms too high. Your arms cannot help your legs move when the arms are held too high. High, tight arms also lead to excessive rotation in your torso, which reduces your running efficiency.
- Don't carry your arms too low, because they won't help you way down there either.
- Don't swing your elbows out too wide, since this wastes energy and also causes you to twist too much from your trunk.

Posture

One of the biggest mistakes beginners make is to employ poor posture when they run. One common mistake is to lean excessively. Unless you're racing the 200 meters (or shorter), don't lean too far forward. Doing so throws off your balance and leads to overworking your back and thigh muscles.

Proper posture begins with the correct body angle. To get a sense of this body angle, stand up straight against a wall. Your core should be engaged, your chest should be up but not out, your shoulders relaxed, and your buttocks pushed firmly back. Now lean slightly forward from your ankles so that your shoulder blades lift away from the wall. This is the posture with which you should run. It allows for proper breathing, prevents you from overleaning, helps you to lengthen your stride, and makes knee lift easier. Good posture ties your whole body together. It even helps you to have a more efficient footstrike.

In thinking about your posture as you run, you should consider where your hips are when your foot hits the ground. The optimal foot placement occurs when your foot strikes the ground under the center of gravity of your body. A line from your ear through your shoulder and hip should end up at your ankle. You should run with a straight posture and a *slight* forward lean. Look ahead to where you are going, or look at the ground 10–20 feet in front of you.

FACT

An Austrian actor named F. M. Alexander, who lost his voice because he was clenching his throat muscles, developed a posture-enhancing technique known today the world over as the Alexander Technique. Beneficial for anyone from daylong computer users to professional athletes, the Alexander Technique, by helping you become more aware of your posture, takes stress off your body and enables you to move more freely.

As you are running also be careful not to stick out your chest, since doing so increases tension in the muscles in your upper back and neck. Your shoulders should be relaxed and your core engaged. Even as you focus on good posture, remember to relax. You want to run standing up straight, but comfortably so.

The Mechanics of Running Hills

Running on level ground requires somewhat different mechanics than going up and down hills. What benefits a long-distance runner on flat ground can fail you in negotiating hills successfully. One of the few good things about hills is that they force you to use muscles you don't normally use, and, if you're fortunate, you get to run as many downhills as uphills.

Running Uphill

Even though you won't be able to maintain the same speed running uphill as you do on the flats, try to maintain the same effort level. Exaggerate your armswing to assist your legs. Imagine that you are cranking your way up or pulling yourself up the hill using your upper body. Shorten your stride, lift your knees higher, lean slightly into the hill, and power on up.

Running Downhill

One of the best things about running downhill is that you can use gravity to your advantage. It is a valuable running skill to learn how to negotiate a downhill effectively without losing control or wasting energy by holding back your speed too much. Although your natural tendency is to lean back when going downhill, you should instead lean forward slightly to maintain a posture in relation to the ground, as if you were running on the flat. Try to keep your footstrike light so as not to grind your heels into the hill as a braking mechanism. Use upper body positioning (leaning) to make speed and body balance adjustments relative to how steep a grade you are running down.

Runners with little prior experience with downhill running should be careful. The biggest risk of injury is to your knees and quads. By catching your "controlled fall," your quadriceps do the bulk of the work of braking. On long downhill stretches, your quads can be overworked without your being aware of it.

If you are racing in a short race, you may lean forward a bit and fly down the hill, but certainly be more careful in training. In fact, many runners who use hills as part of their advanced training either walk or lightly jog down a hill to recover before charging up again. This is a good way to rest and recover while avoiding the excessive knee stress that downhill running can cause.

CHAPTER 7

Cross-Training and Weight Training

Cross-training is an important part of running. By challenging your muscles in new and unique ways, cross-training prevents you from falling into a training rut, and can increase your fitness gains. Weight training, like cross-training, can enhance your running by both improving your performance and reducing your chances of incurring injury. By incorporating weight training into your exercise regimen, you can improve your running performance by increasing abdominal, back, arm, and leg strength. This chapter examines how to incorporate both of these valuable practices into your running routine.

Cross-Training

Although cross-training provides numerous benefits, too much of a good thing can be counterproductive and detrimental to your running. For example, partaking of certain cross-training activities on a scheduled rest day can leave you tired prior to an important workout, such as a long run (especially if you're in training for a half-marathon or marathon).

Furthermore, engaging in certain cross-training activities can actually increase the likelihood of an injury, particularly during the mileage buildup stage. This, in turn, can prevent you from completing the training necessary to attain your goal of finishing a distance event, from a 5K to a marathon. After learning from this chapter about which cross-training activities are beneficial for running, choose your cross-training activities carefully and schedule those sessions to enhance rather than detract from your running goals.

Benefits and Purposes of Cross-Training

Some of the great benefits of cross-training are that it adds variety to your training and decreases the chances of burnout. Also, certain activities, such as cycling, strengthen running-related muscle groups and soft connective tissue, and so help to prevent running injury. You can occasionally substitute cross-training for easy-day running as an aerobic workout.

Cross-training, of course, provides an extra way to burn fat. Many cross-training activities, such as rowing or using a climbing wall, increase upper body strength. Upper body strength is very important in races of all distances, since neck and shoulder muscles often become fatigued. Upper body strength is also important for running uphill.

Precautions and Considerations

Remember, cross-training is not intended to replace running but rather to supplement and enhance it. According to the concept of sports specificity, in order to excel in a particular sport or activity, you must train your muscles and body systems by participating in that specific activity. A 90-minute bike ride can't substitute for a 90-minute run because bike riding doesn't provide the same training effect as running. The bike riding has benefit, however, as it can improve your overall cardiovascular endurance and strengthen your leg muscles with less impact stresses on your legs.

ALERT

Use common sense when deciding whether to add a particular sport to your fitness regimen. Avoid high-impact fitness routines, especially those with quick or sudden movements. Don't participate strenuously in sports in which quick movements can traumatize the soft connective tissue that surrounds the knees and ankles.

Sudden strains or tears resulting from just a fun pickup game can seriously sideline your running goals, so if you've been putting in training time for a big race, why risk it? Also avoid high-impact sports with quick or sudden movements like tennis, racquetball, basketball, soccer, volleyball, downhill skiing, kick-boxing, and aerobic dance.

Ideal Cross-Training Activities

The following are cross-training activities ideally suited to enhance your running performance. They are recommended because they are all "north-south exercises," which place little side-to-side lateral pressures on your body, especially on your leg joints, muscles, and connective tissue. Although these cross-training activities offer good cardiovascular workouts, they also give the legs a heavy-duty workout and therefore should not be done on scheduled leg rest days.

Cycling

Cycling exercises some of the same muscle groups as running, such as the quadriceps, which don't develop as rapidly from workouts as the calf muscles and hamstrings do. Cycling also strengthens the connective tissue of the knee, hip, and ankle regions, thus reducing the risk of injury. After a stressful run, an easy cycling session can loosen fatigued leg muscles.

There are three types of biking to try: road riding, mountain biking, and stationary cycling. Road biking allows you to travel long distances with speed. Mountain bikes are two-wheel, all-terrain vehicles that can be ridden almost anywhere. Although mountain biking is a lot of fun and is challenging, its jarring nature makes falls risky. Road and stationary cycling are better alternatives. With stationary cycling, you can work out indoors year-round regardless of inclement weather. Stationary cycling offers the additional benefit of being able to safely listen to music or read while working out.

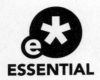

ESSENTIAL

Remember these cycling tips: First, always maintain control when riding your bike. To slow down or stop, *feather* the brakes—alternate between squeezing and releasing them. Also, be aware of cars; don't assume that drivers see you. When you ride past parked cars, watch for car doors opening suddenly. Observe traffic signals and signs, and use hand signals to indicate turns or stops.

A few things to keep in mind: Refrain from cycling on a scheduled rest day. Since it's much more difficult to run after cycling, run prior to heading out on your bike. Spin easily at 80–90 pedal revolutions per minute, as opposed to grinding big gears. Be sure that your seat height and pedals are properly positioned. Finally, always wear a helmet, and leave the iPod at home!

Water Activities

For the compulsive athlete, swimming is one of the best cross-training activities to add to your running regimen. Swimming gives tired leg muscles a breather while providing an excellent upper body workout. Additionally, water has a therapeutic effect on all muscle groups. Although gentle kicking alleviates some muscle soreness and fatigue, avoid using the kickboard for hard kick sets on your running rest day.

If you swim for the aerobic benefit, do not be concerned that your heart rate does not get as high as during other activities. The loss of gravitational force, the horizontal position, and the cooling effect of the water temperature all contribute toward keeping your heart rate low. A general rule is that the swimming heart rate is typically ten to twenty beats per minute less than that for dry land activities.

Another type of water cross-training activity is deep-water running. In deep-water running, you are suspended vertically in a pool by wearing a flotation belt around your waist or a vest around your torso. You simulate running in place in the water without your feet touching the bottom of the pool.

Because there is no shock from footstrike, deep-water running is a perfect alternative to a midweek easy-day run.

Exercise Machines

One of the most-widely used machines in the gym these days is the elliptical trainer. Offering a total-body cardiovascular workout, its elliptical motion combines the effects of classic cross-country skiing, stair climbing, and walking without any pounding of the joints. You can program the elliptical trainer to operate forward, backward, or in a combination of motions, providing a low-impact workout for all the major muscles in the legs. The backward motion emphasizes the *gluteal* muscles (buttocks). You can achieve a good upper body workout by grasping the two arms located on either side of the machine in conjunction with leg motion.

A non-impact cross-training machine gaining in popularity at many gyms is the Cybex® Arc Trainer®. The Arc Trainer® is manufactured with two basic designs for hand placement. Some models are manufactured with side arms that are grasped with the hands and swivel in conjunction with leg motion, providing a total-body workout. The other design has stationary rails, rather than arms, that the user grasps for stability, making it more of a lower-body machine. Offering broad incline and resistance ranges along with numerous programs from which to choose, the intensity of Arc Trainer® workouts can be highly varied. The lower incline levels provide a gliding experience, similar to that of cross-country skiing, while the midrange levels provide a striding effect, much like that of an elliptical trainer. At the upper levels, the Arc Trainer® provides the feel of a stepper or climber machine.

Still found at some gyms are stepper machines, which strengthen and tone the legs while providing a cardiovascular workout. The two basic types are the stair-climber and step mill.

The stair-climber is made of two foot plates that are pushed down, mimicking the effect of climbing up stairs. Because you are working against gravity and body weight, these machines can be hard on the knees. The step mill functions like a revolving staircase or never-ending escalator, providing an intense cardiovascular workout similar to that of climbing stadium steps. The step mill is not for the beginner, as even at lower speeds it can increase one's heart rate rapidly.

Another popular cross-training machine is the ergometer, or rowing machine. As scullers have known for centuries, rowing is a terrific all-body exercise, strengthening your back, buttocks, and legs, and developing your shoulders and arms. It's important to follow good form on a rowing machine, so make sure you ask your health club to show you how to use it properly.

The climbing wall is another piece of equipment that more and more gyms, community centers, and schools are providing. Climbing provides an excellent total-body workout and is mentally and physically challenging, combining balance with footwork and technique. Gyms with indoor climbing walls have the ropes and equipment you need on hand, so you don't have to invest in them. Although it doesn't give a high-intensity cardiovascular workout, it's another way to stretch your muscles while challenging yourself—and it can be very entertaining.

Weight Training to Enhance Running

Whether you are young or old, heavy or lean, a distance runner or a sprinter, you will benefit from weight training, also called strength training. The increase in lean muscle mass that you build from strength training is key to your overall strength and to your body's ability to burn calories. This is because muscle cells require more energy—and therefore burn more calories—than fat cells.

ALERT

If you have medical problems, such as heart disease, diabetes, or high blood pressure, or if you are over forty, be cleared by your doctor before you begin strength training. If you have carpal tunnel syndrome or any other upper extremity physical problem, you should also consult your physician prior to beginning any strength training program.

After the age of thirty, people's muscle mass and metabolism gradually begin to diminish. As this occurs, people find that they can no longer eat all they used to without gaining body fat. You may weigh less at age forty-five than you did at thirty-five, but body composition testing might indicate that you are carrying less muscle and more body fat than you did at a younger age. Incorporating strength training three times or so per week in your training schedule can slow this process considerably.

Overall fitness requires more than just cardiovascular fitness. A balance of endurance, strength, and flexibility must be achieved. The components of fitness include:

- Muscular strength and muscular endurance
- Flexibility
- Cardiovascular endurance
- Body composition

Upper Body Benefits of Weight Training

A strong upper body enables a runner to maintain form late in a marathon or a long run. Additionally, upper body strength reduces fatigue and stiffness in the arms, shoulders, and neck areas. Strong arms and shoulders are helpful in propelling a runner uphill. Finally, legs move only as fast as the arms swing. Thus, a runner with a strong upper body runs faster and more efficiently.

Lower Body Benefits of Weight Training

Running can create a muscular imbalance in the legs. Through running, your quads and calf muscles can become stronger than your hamstrings and shin muscles. Weight training helps address this imbalance. Additionally, strong quadriceps and hips help protect these areas from a variety of injuries. Strong legs also offer some injury protection when running fast downhill.

Other Benefits of Weight Training

Weight training also helps protect bones. This is an important benefit, particularly for menopausal women, because decreased estrogen production causes bone demineralization, which in turn increases the risk of osteoporosis and stress fractures. The pulling action of muscle attachments on bone that happens during weight training facilitates bone regeneration.

Weight training may also help prevent some life-threatening illnesses. Some studies suggest that strength training may reduce the risk factors for adult-onset diabetes and heart disease.

Upper Body Versus Lower Body

Although many athletes train their entire body with equal intensity and use heavy weights for their legs, heavy strength training for the legs is neither necessary nor helpful for the distance runner. Elite athletes and advanced competitive runners engage in strength training that emphasizes the upper body during their training. Following their example, go easy on the legs, using strength training cautiously (using low weights with a high number of repetitions) while emphasizing upper body work.

Some runners, who begin losing muscle mass as they age, find that lower extremity exercises are helpful in maintaining their strength. Some younger runners then assume that if more strength is good for the aging athlete, then it must be good for the younger one too. This, however, is not necessarily so. Younger athletes are not losing muscle mass by 5–20 percent while they are still in their prime. Young runners are best off performing only light lower-body strengthening in combination with a varied training regimen that includes workouts and drills to enhance their running speed, form, and strength. Such workouts include fartlek ("speed play") workouts, striders, hill repeats, tempo runs, and repeat intervals.

Of course, there is still value in performing graded leg presses, leg curls, hip abduction exercises, straight leg lifts, calf raises, and core strengthening exercises. Just don't go overboard on strengthening the muscles that runners exercise the most.

Practical Weight Training

Since this is a running book, the weight training exercises included here are ones that you can do at home and that give you all the benefits described above. Although these exercises don't require that you go to the gym, if you want to take this training to the next level, go for it! Work with someone knowledgeable at the gym so you are using the appropriate amount of weight to work the muscles you want to target. And remember what was said about overworking your legs—it's not a good idea.

Types of Weights to Use

If you're starting as a complete beginner, the best weights to use for upper body strengthening are dumbbells, which you can buy at a sporting goods store. Dumbbells are convenient, portable, and not overwhelming. You can use them while watching television or talking on the phone. They come in various weights, and you'll need a few so you can use different dumbbells to work different muscles. If the only upper body work you've done is lifting utensils to eat and lifting a glass (or mug) to drink, you probably want to start out with 3-pound weights. You'll graduate to 5 pounds in a few weeks and may be ready to work with 8- to 10-pound weights in a few months.

You may also want to purchase weights for lower body work. A handy type of weight to use for leg strengthening is a cuff weight that goes around your ankle and attaches with a Velcro® strap. Again, be sure not to overdo it with leg exercises!

Using Weights

There are two ways to hold your dumbbells: overhand and underhand. For the overhand grip, grab the dumbbell with your palm facing downward. For the underhand grip, your palm should be facing upward.

There are at least two ways to stand as well. One is with your feet shoulder-width apart, head and shoulders level, back erect, and knees slightly bent. This is the standard stance. Another position is bent over, feet shoulder-width apart, with one leg slightly extended. The idea is to work with a flat back and with your nonworking arm resting on the same-side thigh (for a level surface).

When first beginning a strength training program, you should only perform one set of each exercise for the first couple of weeks, doing twelve to fifteen repetitions (reps) of an exercise. Don't feel overwhelmed and think you must increase the number of sets to reap strength training benefits. After this you may increase to two or three sets after one warm-up set. If you feel as if you could go well beyond fifteen to twenty reps, increase the weight on your next set or at your next session.

Upper Body Exercises

Your upper body workout should target the upper body muscles described above. Remember, for maximum results, use the appropriate weight (the weight at which you can do no more than twelve to fifteen reps).

Biceps Curl and Triceps Kickback

From the standing position, arms at your sides, hold a 3- to 5-pound dumbbell with an underhand grip. With your elbow securely against your side, raise (curl) the dumbbell up and toward your chest as far as it will go, and then control the weight as you bring your hand back down. This is one repetition. Alternate arms after each set.

For the triceps kickback, use an overhand grip on a 3- to 5-pound dumbbell and, standing in the bent-over position, extend the working arm straight back behind you (kick it back) without completely extending your elbow. Control the weight as you bend your arm back toward your chest. This is one repetition.

Front Raise and Shoulder Press

The *front raise* works your deltoids. In the standing position, with a 3- to 5-pound dumbbell in an overhand grip, let both arms rest in front of your body so that your palms are resting on your thighs. Lift one arm straight up to shoulder height, keeping your elbow straight so that your arm is parallel to the floor. Control the weight on the way back to the starting position for one repetition.

For the *shoulder press*, stand with the dumbbells in an overhand grip, bend your arms so that the dumbbells are by your ears, palms facing away from your body. Press the dumbbell up over your head, and then lower the weight to the starting position for one rep.

Bent-Over Row

From the bent-over position, hold a 5- to 10-pound dumbbell in an overhand grip and extend your arm toward the floor in a diagonal line from your shoulder. As if you were rowing a boat, bend your elbow and lift the dumbbell in a slow, smooth circular motion so that you use your mid-back muscles as well as your arm muscles. Return to the starting position for one rep.

Lower Body Exercises

These exercises target your major lower body muscles. Keep in mind that as a runner you don't want to overwork your legs, which get a workout every time you run.

Lunges

Stand with feet shoulder-width apart, and a 5- to 10-pound dumbbell in each hand in the overhand grip. Step out with your right leg about one stride, landing on your heel and rolling your foot down flat against the floor. Bend both knees so that your right thigh is parallel to the floor; do not let your right knee go beyond your right foot. Your left thigh will be perpendicular to it, and your left heel will lift off the floor. Your arms remain by your sides during the exercise. Return to the starting position by rolling off the ball of your right foot. Alternate legs as you do your reps.

Leg Extensions

Sit in a chair with firm back support and your feet resting flat on the floor. Attach a 5- to 10-pound cuff weight to each ankle. One leg at a time, lift your leg until your knee is straight. Control the descent. This is one rep.

Leg Curls

Lie face down on the floor, with your arms at your side and a 5- to 10-pound cuff weight on each ankle. Turn your head to one side and lift both feet toward your buttocks, bringing your heels as close to your buttocks as you can. Use your abs to keep your hips pressing into the floor and lower your legs to the starting position for one rep.

Exercises for Abs and Back

Use the following exercises to strengthen your abdominal and back muscles. You can do some of these every day, so long as you don't overdo it.

Pelvic Tilt

Lying on your back on the floor, preferably on a mat or folded towel for some cushion, bend your knees, rest your heels on the floor, and let your toes point up. Keep your arms at your side. Imagine gravity pulling your bellybutton onto the floor so that your lower back is flattened against the floor. This will cause your pelvis to rise slightly, and you should feel your abs tighten. Do not push through your legs—use only your abdominal muscles to flatten your back. Hold this position for several seconds, then relax and repeat. Do three sets of ten reps.

Abdominal Crunch

Lie on your back with your knees bent and feet flat on the floor, about shoulder-width part. Bring your arms up and put your hands behind your head, thumbs pointing toward your ears. Don't interlock your fingers, even if your fingers overlap. Keep your head extended from your body so that your chin isn't digging into your chest. Start raising your trunk, curling up from your spine, and using your abs—not your hands—to pull yourself up.

ESSENTIAL

Rather than lifting heavy weights only a few times like bodybuilders and power lifters do, emphasize lighter weights and more repetitions (twelve to fifteen). Don't overdo exercises that might leave your legs fatigued for your next run. Instead, concentrate your efforts on your upper body and carefully choose the lower extremity exercises that work for you.

Keep your elbows to the side and raise yourself up only enough to lift your shoulder blades off the floor. Pause, and then bring your trunk back into position slowly for one repetition. Start by doing three sets of fifteen reps, adjusting according to whether it feels like too much or not enough.

After you're in better shape, you can increase the intensity of your ab crunch workout: Try doing your reps with your legs off the floor, crossed at your ankles. Keep your knees bent and your butt on the floor.

Weight-Training Tips

For a successful weight-training experience, keep the following guidelines in mind:

- Warm up before lifting, and stretch thoroughly afterward.
- Run prior to lifting, and avoid weight training leg work on days before races, speed workouts, or long runs.
- Lift every other day or three days per week.
- Emphasize lighter weights and more repetitions rather than heavy weights with few reps.
- Don't hold your breath while lifting weights; breathe in on the relaxation phase and out while performing the hard part of the exercise.
- Move your joint through its entire range of motion when lifting a weight, making sure you don't lock your joints while performing the exercise.
- Follow the sequence of legs first, upper body second, and midsection last, remembering to work your abdominal muscles.
- In each sequence, exercise the larger muscle groups first, followed by the smaller groups.

FACT

Remember, you probably won't lose weight as you incorporate a weight-conditioning program into your present training. Instead, you will gain muscle and lower body fat (assuming you eat sensibly). Thus the bathroom scale can be very misleading. Although your weight may not change, as you lose fat and gain muscle, your clothes will fit better, and you'll look and feel great!

Run First, Lift Later

It is best for runners to run first and do strength training second, preferably not back-to-back. If possible, schedule several hours between a run and your strength workout. You may run in the morning and then do your strength routine at lunchtime or in the evening. If you are forced to perform the two routines together, do your run first and then your strength training. If you are doing a long run or a speed workout, hold off on the strength training afterward. You'll probably be too tired to perform it properly.

Some have recommended that you perform your hard running and strength training on the same day (but separate the two), followed by an easy run the next day so you have time to recover. Experiment to see what feels right to you. You might find it easier to do your strength training on a light running day or even on a rest day. For more advanced runners, if you do strength training on a rest day, go very easy on the legs or skip the leg workouts entirely if you will be racing or doing a speed-work session the next day.

CHAPTER 8

On the Road to Speed

How can you increase your speed? Most runners ask this question once they become more accomplished. Indeed, one of the best things about running is being able to compete not only against others but also against yourself. Improvement is almost always possible, but it is also dependent upon so many factors, including one's age, current fitness level, genetics, experience level, type of training program, motivation, etc. If you run faster this week, can you run even faster next? This chapter gives you insight into adding speed work to your workout.

Adding Speed Work

Incorporating some carefully designed faster-paced runs is essential to a program seeking faster performance in your daily training runs and in races you enter. For the more accomplished runner, incorporating some advanced running techniques is necessary to improve your time from one race to the next. Your best race times are referred to as PRs (personal records) or PBs (personal bests).

FACT

PR (personal record) and PB (personal best) both represent your fastest time posted at a given distance. In order to claim a PR or PB, you should perform on a track or a road race course certified as accurate by USA Track & Field (USATF), the national governing body for track and field, long-distance running, and race walking.

If you are new to running, don't entertain the notion of adding speed work to your training regimen until you have been running regularly (logging 20–25 miles per week) for at least a year. Running speed workouts without this solid mileage base greatly increases your chances of incurring an injury. If you do decide to focus on this aspect of your running, it is important to read this entire section before beginning any speed workout on your own.

The Risks

Despite the benefits of increasing your speed, incorporating advanced training techniques into your regimen exponentially increases your risk of injury. You really need to think about whether you are willing, after months of training, to risk injury that prevents you from participating in your chosen events. A mistake here can result in serious, if not languorous, injuries that can keep you from running for weeks or even months at a time.

The Benefits

The physical gains attained through speed work are more numerous than you might think. There's the obvious, which of course is improved strength and speed. However, these are actually by-products of the training. With higher-intensity training, you now have a better oxygen delivery system. You can run faster and still stay at a comfortable aerobic (meaning, using oxygen as fuel) pace. Your body becomes more efficient at delivering oxygen to your muscles, and your muscles function better while using less oxygen.

When you run at a faster and faster pace, your body reaches the point where it exceeds its capacity to use oxygen as fuel and you begin using glycogen (a carbohydrate) as your primary fuel source. The point at which you cross over from aerobic to anaerobic (without oxygen) systems is called the *anaerobic threshold*. A by-product of using this anaerobic system for energy production is lactic acid.

Advanced running techniques can raise your anaerobic threshold, thereby delaying the onset of oxygen debt. Oxygen debt—that heavy, burning feeling in your legs that makes your muscles tie up—is caused by a buildup of lactic acid. With specific anaerobic training, you can run at a faster pace before you reach your anaerobic threshold. This, in turn, will improve your running times.

Mental Edge

The mental benefits of doing speed work result from your setting and achieving time-related goals. Running PRs off your improved speed is quite fulfilling and can be highly motivating. Speed work can be challenging and sometimes quite uncomfortable, perhaps even painful (not to be confused with the pain associated with injury, however).

You are asking your body to perform faster and outside of the aerobic zone, which through training has become comfortable with long, slow runs. You're pushing the limits of your body and mind, past previous physical and mental barriers. The end result is that your mental toughness improves significantly, both during fast-paced training runs and when competing in races of all distances.

Race Strategy

Last, but certainly not least, you'll benefit from planning and implementing a smart race day strategy. Speed workouts furnish you with improved stamina throughout an entire race, which alone results in a better finish time. A smart race strategy entails planning your race in advance. Rather than sprinting through the first part of a 5K (as if you're competing in the Olympic 100-meter finals) and having little energy left for the rest of the race, your experience from running intervals on a track can give you a good idea of what pace you should run during a race.

Quick Guidelines for Speed Work

Some basic guidelines for speed work are as follows. First, you should be consistently running a minimum of 20–25 miles per week for a year before you even begin to think about including advanced training techniques in your training schedule. Be sure to follow a *hard-easy method of training* if you intend to integrate speed training into your program. For example, do not schedule a speed work session the day after a long run or after participating in a road race. If their longest run of the week is on Sunday, most experienced runners do their speed training during the middle of the week following either an easy run or a complete leg rest day. You could follow a training pattern something like this: Monday HARD, Tuesday EASY, Wednesday HARD, Thursday EASY, Friday EASY (or off), Saturday RACE or LONG, Sunday EASY.

If you choose to participate in speed work with a group, be sure to run at a pace appropriate for your ability level. Trying to perform a workout designed for someone else greatly increases your chances of incurring an injury and can also be discouraging. To avoid injury, proper warm-ups and cool-downs are essential. These include light jogging followed by stretching both before and after the workout.

No more than 15–20 percent of your total weekly mileage should be fast-paced running. This percentage covers both speed workouts and races. You should not increase the volume of your fast-paced running by more than 800 meters per week.

If you elect to do speed workouts during the summer months, schedule them for the early morning or in the evening to avoid the hottest and most humid times of the day. Pushing the pace in such conditions increases your chances of suffering from heat illness.

Finally, be careful of what you eat and how late you time your meal or snack before fast-paced running. Experimenting with a variety of food and drink is the best way to determine what your system can tolerate. Don't eat a big lunch if you're planning on doing a fast-paced run later in the afternoon. Instead, have small snacks throughout the day.

ESSENTIAL

One of the best ways to find others who do speed work in your area is to contact a local running club. You can find a running club by contacting the Road Runners Club of America (*www.rrca.org*) for a list of running clubs throughout the nation. Many running clubs hold weekly speed workout sessions at a local track and sometimes offer seminars at club meetings.

Hill Repeats

As the name suggests, hill repeats are repetitive charges—running fast-paced efforts up hills. Integrate hill repeats (considered a strengthening workout) into your training schedule after the base-building stage. This will be the time period when you slowly and carefully build weekly mileage levels (with increases of no more than 10 percent per week).

Hill repeats are also an excellent means to prepare your leg strength and cardiovascular system for the rest of the advanced workouts. Besides deriving benefits from strengthening your legs, hill repeats enhance your mental toughness for workouts and races on hilly terrain. Although you may never gain an unconditional love for hill training or racing on hilly courses, you will at least face challenging terrains with confidence.

Practicing Hill Repeats

After a warm-up jog of 1–1½ miles (or a minimum of 12 minutes of easy running), assault the hill at 5K effort pace (that's effort, not speed). The idea is to aggressively run up the hill while maintaining good running form.

As you reach the end point of the uphill section (generally, 100 meters for the novice and up to 200 meters for the experienced runner), your breathing should feel very labored and your legs quite heavy. Turn around and jog (or walk) very easily down the hill, then continue on flat ground for 30 meters or so before turning around for the next repeat.

Depending on your level of experience and fitness, the number of repeats will vary. The novice should do no more than four repeats the first week, adding two additional repeats each week for the next three to four weeks. The experienced runner can begin with six repeats and proceed from there. As with any workout, it is important to cool down by jogging at least a mile (or a minimum of 10–12 minutes) afterward.

HILL REPEAT BASICS

- Shorten your stride
- Lean slightly into the hill
- Keep your head up, focusing on what's just in front of you rather than on the top of the hill or incline
- Maintain a consistent effort up the hill
- Swing your arms (up and down rather than side to side)
- Stay mentally focused and self-directed, pushing forward until you complete the hill repeat

Fartlek, or "Speed Play," Workouts

Fartlek, a Swedish word meaning "speed play," is an unstructured type of speed work. The central purpose of fartlek runs is to train you for the anaerobic demands that more structured speed workouts and racing provide. Whereas more structured speed workouts, generally done on a track or an accurately measured course, encompass specified periods and distances of fast-paced running followed by recovery periods, the fartlek workout is quite different. You can run a fartlek workout at a fast pace in varying distances and durations.

Fartlek Running Guidelines

Even though it is considered an unstructured workout, there are basic guidelines for fartlek running. Begin your workout with a minimum of 1–1½ miles of easy running (or a minimum of 12 minutes). End with a 1-mile cool-down, throw in speed bursts of varying times and distances, and then follow each with a recovery jog. The idea here is to practice running at a brisk effort (generally faster than your present 5K race pace), employing good running form and training your body to run anaerobically (meaning, without oxygen). Push yourself until your breathing becomes labored and your pace begins to drop off.

ALERT

Just as you can run fartlek workouts in a variety of ways, you can perform them on various terrains, including on roads and trails. Before doing fartleks on hilly courses, however, it's best to accustom yourself to these workouts by running them on flat ground.

Planning a Fartlek Workout

So as not to overdo exercise and risk incurring an overuse injury, you should develop a specific plan for incorporating fartlek workouts into your training program. The first week the novice might aim for 4 minutes of total fast-paced running (for example, 30 seconds + 30 seconds + 30 seconds + 45 seconds + 45 seconds + 30 seconds + 30 seconds), adding 2 minutes of fast effort for each of the next three weeks. By having a specific plan ahead of time for enduring a cumulation of fast periods of running, you are less likely to risk injury by overdoing your workout.

Striders and Tempo Runs

Also known as "pickups," striders are generally done following your warm-up jog prior to the beginning of an interval session or a road race to prepare your legs and cardiovascular system for the fast-paced running to immediately follow. The distance of striders is approximately 80 meters. These are best run on a straightaway rather than around curves. Begin by gradually increasing your pace so that you're running with a full stride (but not at full speed) by the 30- to 40-meter mark. Hold the pace for the next 10 meters before gradually reducing your speed to a jog by the end of the 80 meters.

The purpose of the strider is to achieve a long, full-stride length at a comfortable speed. You do not want to sprint all out in a strider. Turn around and repeat this process four times (for a beginner) to ten times (for an advanced competitor). Time your striders so that your speed workout or race follows a couple of minutes later.

Tempo Runs

The primary purpose of including tempo runs in your regimen is to increase your anaerobic threshold to maintain a faster pace over longer periods of time. A secondary purpose of the tempo run is to simulate racing conditions by running at or near your race pace over a distance shorter than the race. The pace of the tempo run should be about 10–15 seconds slower than your present 10K race pace. Depending on your race goals, the tempo segment of your run can be anywhere from 6 continuous minutes to 20 minutes or more.

Rather than doing a structured warm-up that includes stretching and striders, start out your tempo workout by running easily for at least 12 minutes or longer before cruising into the fast segment. An example of a tempo run workout is to run 12 minutes at tempo pace followed by a 6-minute recovery jog. You could then tack on another 12-minute segment at tempo pace before concluding the balance of your workout with easy running.

Interval Workouts

Interval workouts consist of a series of short, fast-paced runs, generally a mile or less in distance, separated by recovery jogs. There are many variations of interval workouts, each with its own rationale, but all with a goal of raising your anaerobic threshold and improving your overall speed in race distances from the mile to the marathon.

Prior to beginning any type of interval session, it is very important to begin with a thorough warm-up featuring easy jogging, stretching, and striders. Equally important is the cool-down that concludes the workout.

There are three basic types of interval workouts: repeat intervals, pyramids, and ladders. Each is described below. First, though, some general concepts about intervals need introduction.

The theory behind the interval workout is simple. Let's use a 5K race (3.1 miles) as an example.

First, you determine your present mile pace in a short-distance race such as a 5K. There are several variables in an interval workout that you can tweak to change the level of difficulty. You can adjust the target time for the repeat interval up or down, increase or decrease the recovery (time or distance), or increase or decrease the number of repeats that you run. If you are a novice, an experienced runner or a coach can assist you in designing interval workouts appropriate for both your present ability level and your short- and long-term running goals.

FACT

Interval workouts feature two major components. First, they have a fast-paced segment, called the *repeat,* which is run over a specified distance at a targeted goal time. That is followed by a brief rest period called the *recovery.*

The target time for the repeat interval (the distance of the fast-paced segment) is usually based on your current race pace in a short-race distance such as a 5K. The most common distances for which to practice fast-pace efforts include 200 meters, 400 meters, 600 meters, 800 meters, 1,200 meters, 1,600 meters, and a mile (1,609 meters). Although novices first attempting interval workouts might practice running the shorter segments, such as 400 meters, at their current race pace, more experienced competitors would do these 20–40 seconds per mile faster.

ALERT

The quality of your interval workout is often affected by leg fatigue even before you start the workout. Lack of restorative rest or not warming up properly can leave your legs feeling heavy and weak. You might require a longer warm-up jog or more stretching. Environmental conditions such as warm temperatures and high humidity or stiff headwinds also can negatively affect your performance during these fast-paced workouts.

For the experienced runner, the recovery jog following the repeat is typically either half the distance or twice the time of the interval you run. For example, if you just ran 400 meters in 90 seconds, you could either do a recovery jog of 200 meters (half the distance) or for 3 minutes (twice the time). The novice first attempting these workouts should allow a longer recovery period, however.

Repeat Intervals

These are workouts in which the distance of the fast-paced segment remains constant. For example, the workout could feature six 400-meter repeats with a 200-meter recovery jog after each, or four 800-meter repeats each followed by a 400-meter recovery jog after each.

It is important to run consistent times for the repeats. You should try to run the final repeat in approximately the same time as you ran the first. The goal is not to run until you collapse, but to maintain your form and target pace throughout the workout. The idea here is to leave the track feeling that, if you wanted to, you could do one or two more repeat intervals.

If you find that your speed really falls off after the first couple of repeats, your target time for these may be too fast for your current level of conditioning. You can either adjust the workout from the original plan by increasing your goal times for the repeats (running the repeats at a slower pace), allow yourself more recovery between the fast-paced segments, or bag the workout entirely and attempt it another day.

FACT

Abbreviations are often used in books, magazine articles, or by coaches to describe specific speed workouts. For example: 6 × 400M in 1:40, 200R means that you will be asked to run six 400-meter repeats (once around the track) in 1 minute and 40 seconds, followed by a 200-meter recovery jog after each of the repeats.

Pyramids and Ladders

Pyramids and ladders are also considered part of the interval family. Rather than running the same distances for all your repeat intervals, you vary the length of each, running longer or shorter repeats throughout the workout. Pyramid workouts feature fast segments increasing and then decreasing in distance. For example, your fast segments could progress upward from 200 to 400 meters and topping out at 800 meters before going down again to 400 and then 200 meters. As is the case with repeat intervals, a recovery period of easy jogging follows each of the fast-paced segments during a pyramid or ladder workout.

A ladder is a progression either up or down in repeat interval length. For example, your repeats could progress upward with longer and longer lengths: 200 meters, followed by 400, 800, 1,200, and ending with 1,600 meters. Or you could run the ladder workout in reverse order beginning with the longest distance of your fast-paced segments (1,600, 1,200, 800, 400, 200 meters).

Important Warm-Up and Cool-Down Procedures

With the exception of fartlek and tempo runs (during which you will be doing some easy jogging prior to rolling into their fast-paced segments), it is important to develop a regular warm-up routine you can use for every interval workout and race you do. The warm-up is important for three reasons. First of all, running at a fast pace without a proper warm-up greatly increases your chances of incurring an injury. Second, your muscles perform more efficiently and optimally after being properly warmed up. Third, following a consistent routine decreases the anxiety and stress that sometimes precede difficult workouts and races.

Your Warm-Up Routine

It is very important to plan for and allow adequate time for your warm-up so that you're not rushed getting to the starting line of a race or to begin a speed workout session. Begin your warm-up with a minimum of 12 minutes of easy jogging. When you are racing shorter distances (such as the 5K) or when the weather is cold, you may want to increase the time or distance of your warm-up jog.

Next, you want to stretch all your major leg muscles (calves, hamstrings, quads, hips) thoroughly for several minutes. Again, don't rush yourself!

While stretching, take a few swigs of water to top off your reservoir. It's better to hydrate at this time so as to have an effective speed workout without interruption. If it's a warm day, however, use common sense and drink fluids as often as conditions dictate.

The last event prior to your speed workout or race is to run four to ten striders of 80 meters, as described earlier. After completing these, take a minute or two to catch your breath. You are now prepared to run hard.

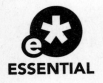

ESSENTIAL

Rather than running lap after lap on a track (which can be quite boring), do your warm-up on a road or a grass field. Spare your knees, ankles, and hips the unnecessary wear and tear resulting from frequent turns on a track.

Your Cool-Down Routine

Don't consider your workout or race over until you cool down properly. Even when performing your daily runs at a comfortable pace, you should finish up a workout by jogging easily the last 10 minutes and then stretch immediately afterward.

After running a race or hard workout, it is even more important to jog easily for 10 minutes or longer so that your breathing and heart rate can return to normal. Following your cool-down jog, invest 10–15 minutes in stretching your major leg muscles (along with any upper body parts that feel tight) thoroughly before calling it quits. By cooling down properly, your muscles recover effectively from hard workout or race demands. Compared with the runner who rushes through or skips his cool-down, you will find that your muscles feel much less stiff, sore, and fatigued later in the day.

Some of the more advanced runners who want to maintain their leg speed while increasing their weekly mileage can run striders following their long runs. As part of your cool down, run eight to ten striders after the run and before stretching.

Speed-Work Programs Based on Experience

When developing a program that integrates advanced training techniques, it is important to remember that there is no "one size fits all" approach. Programs must be individualized to meet your present ability level as well as your goals and needs. This section provides a wide range of essential guidelines, both for the runner first attempting speed work and for the accomplished runner.

ALERT

If you are a beginner or novice attempting speed work for the first time, do not jump ahead and attempt workouts designed for an experienced runner. Injury is almost guaranteed! Progress comes with consistent training over months and years. Train only at your present ability level!

The Beginner

The beginner is the person who has just started a running program within the past year. As emphasized previously, a beginner's primary focus is to build a running base of 20–25 miles per week for a year. By exercising patience during this time, you will strengthen your leg muscles and toughen up your connective tissue to later handle the rigors of more advanced training. A beginner pushing his limits by doing speed workouts before leg muscles have strengthened adequately greatly increases the risk of injury.

Rather than including advanced training techniques in their programs, it's perfectly fine for beginners to enter distance races of 5K and 10K once a month or so for fun and that way gain experience from running in an organized and competitive forum. By occasionally participating in road races, beginners gather an understanding of their present ability level (race pace).

The Novice

A novice runner is one who has consistently been running 20–25 miles per week for a year or more. After this base-building phase, novices can add some advanced training techniques to their training schedules.

This next phase can begin by performing four weeks of hill repeats one time per week. Novices can start with four repeats up a 5 percent grade of 100 meters long, adding two repeats for each of the next three weeks. (Refer to the hill repeat section in this chapter for guidelines.)

You can then engage in fartlek runs during the next four weeks as a transition from the hill-repeat phase to interval training. The novice should begin with 4 minutes of cumulative fast-paced efforts one time per week and increase the duration by 2 minutes each week for the next three weeks. (Please refer to the fartlek section in this chapter for additional guidelines.)

Following eight combined weeks of hill-repeat and fartlek workouts, novices are now ready to include more structured speed work in their training over the next six weeks. Replace the fartlek workout with repeat intervals. Although there are a myriad of options regarding workouts, one plan is to alternate weekly speed sessions between 400-meter and 800-meter repeats. Shoot for running a total of 1½–2 miles worth of intervals altogether. For either workout, be sure not to increase the distance of fast-paced running by more than a total of 800 meters per week. The speed of these repeats should be at the novice's current race pace. A recovery jog between each repeat should be equal to the distance of the repeat. That is, for 400-meter repeats, recovery jogs of 400 meters should be performed between the repeats.

Every third or fourth week, you can enter a 5K or 10K race to evaluate your training progress. Determine your race pace by checking the split times at each mile mark, or calculate your average mile pace from your overall finish time. You can then adjust the speed of future repeat intervals accordingly to allow for continued improvement.

Now is the time to tackle a target race. It is recommended that you taper the final week before the race by cutting your weekly mileage in half. Throw in a few 30-second bursts of speed to top off training during the last speed work session three to four days before the big event. During the race, focus on running an even but aggressive pace that you can maintain throughout the entire race. Turn on the afterburners during the last 800 meters, and try to pass as many runners as possible while maintaining good running form.

Speed Work for the Experienced Runner

Although the base-building guidelines for all runners are the same, the experienced runner may find that she performs best at a level of 40–45 miles per week. Some advanced competitors even log weekly mileage at significantly higher levels. However, lingering leg fatigue and the increased risk of injury can outweigh the gain of running additional mileage per week. Keep in mind that more is not always better, and emphasize running quality over quantity.

Many experienced runners can handle two advanced training workouts per week. Assuming a long run on Sunday, the advanced runner could do a fartlek workout on either Tuesdays or Wednesdays followed by a hill-repeat workout on either Thursdays or Fridays the first four weeks of this phase of training. Listening to your body is the best way to determine which days your legs feel most rested and recovered for these advanced workouts.

For the first week the fartlek workout would encompass 6 minutes of cumulative fast-paced efforts, adding 4 minutes per session for each of the next three weeks. Similarly, the hill repeats would begin with six charges up a 150- to 200-meter incline and adding two repeats per session for each of the next three weeks.

After completing four weeks of fartlek runs and hill repeats, you can begin more formal speed training (interval sessions) and continue these over the next eight to ten weeks. Again, assuming that your long run is Sunday, interval sessions could be performed either on Tuesdays or Wednesdays depending on which day your legs feel most rested. Your present 5K race pace determines how quickly you run these fast segments.

For the sake of this discussion, let's say that your present race pace is 8:00 minutes per mile. In the first week of interval training, aim to run the 400-meter repeats at 7:40 (7 minutes, 40 seconds) pace per mile (1:55 per lap) followed by a 200-meter recovery jog. Repeat this sequence three more times, striving to run a consistent pace for each interval. The next week, run 800 meters at a 7:50 pace per mile (3:55 for two laps) with a 400-meter recovery jog. Repeat this process two more times.

As your speed improves over the course of your racing season, target the 400-meter repeat times to be approximately 20–25 seconds faster than your current 5K race pace. You should run the 800-meter repeats about 10–15 seconds faster than your 5K race pace. By the end of this phase of training, top out weekly interval sessions with workouts of ten to twelve 400-meter repeats and five to six 800-meter repeats. Remember that with any speed workout or race, it is very important to include at least a 1- to 1½-mile warm-up and a 1-mile cool-down jog followed by 10–15 minutes of stretching.

ESSENTIAL

The experienced runner can also vary the interval workouts over the course of the next several weeks, beginning with longer repeat intervals during the earlier part of training (1,600 and 1,200 meters) and shortening the fast-paced segments as the target race gets closer. For variety, also include pyramids and ladder sessions among the possibilities in an interval session.

Along with interval sessions, the experienced runner might also want to include tempo workouts during this period of training. Tempo runs provide an opportunity to practice running at a fast pace for longer periods of time. These could be scheduled two to three days following the interval workout session or occasionally nested within a 10- to 12-mile run. The first week, aim to sustain a swift pace for 6 continuous minutes within the middle part of the workout, adding an additional 4 minutes for each subsequent week. Run the pace of the tempo segment approximately 10–15 seconds per mile slower than your present 10K race pace.

Every third or fourth week, you can substitute a 5K or 10K practice race for a tempo workout or long run to evaluate training progress. From these practice events, determine your current race pace (per mile) and adjust the speed of future repeat interval sessions accordingly to allow for continued improvement.

ALERT

To reduce the strain on your knees (thus minimizing your risk of injury) when running on a track, you can change your running direction midway through your speed workout. This would be especially good to do if you are running on a small indoor track. *Important:* Change directions only if no other runners or walkers are using the track. If you are running the workout with a group, make sure that the other runners also agree to do so.

After the completion of the interval phase of training, you are now ready to race at your optimal level. Through the experience gained over the course of months and years of racing, advanced competitors better understand the maximum level that they can push and maintain their race pace. Unlike the beginner and novice who often measure improvement in minutes, the experienced runner may only be able to improve by a few seconds from race to race.

CHAPTER 9

Barefoot Running

Barefoot running is nothing new. From our earliest roots as hunter-gatherers we ran, and for most of the past 2 million years we likely ran without footwear. It wasn't until the 1970s that the modern running shoe began to correct and control the foot as it does today. So to remove our heavy, high-tech shoes and run barefoot is an old idea, not a new one. Barefoot running and minimalist-shoes running are not for everyone, but they can be either a good supplement to improve your running form and efficiency, or a new method of running in a more natural way while possibly reducing your risk for certain injuries. There is the risk of injury any time you introduce your body to a new sport or activity. If you decide to try barefoot running, a gradual and controlled transition should be made.

What Is Barefoot Running?

Barefoot running is the act of running without shoes on your feet. For much of man's 2 million years of existence, he walked and ran without footwear, or else he wore flimsy sandals or moccasins. Throughout history we have proven ourselves to be well suited for long-distance running.

Dr. Daniel Lieberman and research colleagues at Harvard University studied the biomechanics of endurance running on the body, published their results in January 2010, and share their findings at *http://barefoot running.fas.harvard.edu*. According to Dr. Lieberman, given our body's ability to efficiently disperse heat and our balance of slow- and fast-twitch muscle fibers, humans are the best-adapted endurance runners in the animal kingdom. This ability to run long distances preceded the modern running shoe by a couple of million years. So it stands to reason that we have always been well suited to run without shoes. Indeed, some believe that the human body may be better designed to run without shoes than with them.

If the (Minimalist) Shoe Fits

There are many proponents of barefoot running who believe that the human body was designed to run barefoot. They propose that modern cushioned and supportive running shoes interfere with natural running technique, which results in a greater risk for injury. Others argue that the cushioning and stabilization provided by the modern running shoe are needed to correct weaknesses in form and foot structure to protect runners against overuse injuries. These ongoing debates have clearly not been resolved.

Is Barefoot Running a Fad?

Although it may be too soon to tell, the current barefoot running movement, fueled in part by the success of Christopher McDougall's popular book *Born to Run: A Hidden Tribe, Superathletes, and the Greatest Race the World Has Never Seen*, might be more than a fad. Running the "natural" way has been around for decades but only recently hit the mainstream. The movement within the scientific community is picking up traction as they proclaim the benefits of barefoot or minimalist-shoes running while they disprove the usefulness of the modern high-tech running shoe.

For years many high-level distance runners have made barefoot running part of their training regime. When cushioned, somewhat stiff, and likely overengineered running shoes are worn, the small muscles in your feet and lower legs are not used to control your movement, so they grow relatively weak. The shoes also reduce valuable sensory information from your feet and decrease your *proprioception*—the body's ability to sense and respond to changes in the positions of your foot, ankle, and knee. By running without shoes, you can strengthen the weakened muscles while improving sensory input for balance, proprioception, and form.

FACT

According to Georgia Shaw, marketing manager for Vibram USA, since its popular FiveFingers® line of minimalist running shoes was launched, sales have increased exponentially each year. With the fit like a glove and no cushion or arch support, the FiveFingers® minimalist running footwear is a safer and more comfortable alternative to running completely barefoot.

Fixing Form Flaws

In his book *Natural Running: The Simple Path to Stronger, Healthier Running* (VeloPress, ©2010), Danny Abshire identifies two major running technique mistakes made by distance runners: (1) they land on their heels, which causes a braking of forward momentum and excessive rotational stresses in the leg joints, and (2) they use too much muscle force to create their forward propulsion. These technique flaws lead to excessive vertical oscillation with each stride, which in turn leads to increased impact forces, inefficiency, and unnecessary additional stress on lower extremity muscles and tendons. Additionally, these two form flaws may contribute to some of the most common running overuse injuries, including plantar fasciitis, Achilles tendinitis, shin splints, iliotibial band friction syndrome, and patellofemoral knee pain.

Michael Warburton, PT, MSc, writes that when running on hard surfaces, you compensate for the lack of cushioning from the shoe by landing softer on your feet and by landing on your midfoot rather than on your heel. By landing on your midfoot (or forefoot), the support structures of your feet grow stronger, which will possibly reduce your risk of injury. For example, some believe that barefoot running may reduce the incidence of plantar fasciitis (inflammation of the ligament that runs along the arch of the foot). The job of the plantar fascia when walking or running in shoes is to provide an unyielding support to the longitudinal arch. The lower incidence of plantar fasciitis setbacks in the barefoot running population may be attributed to increased use of associated foot and ankle musculature, which reduces impact forces (and thus the loading stress to the plantar fascia).

ALERT

Stronger muscles in your feet, ankles, and lower legs will also make it easier to land lightly on your midfoot and for your flexed knee to dampen and disperse the forces of impact. Landing on your midfoot will also aid in the elastic recoil provided by your plantar fascia and the tendons and muscles of your foot and lower leg.

Ramping Down

Over the years, running shoes have grown thicker, softer, and heavier. Important sensory input from the foot for proprioception, balance, and form is dampened by the soft materials of the shoes' midsole. The *ramp angle* of the shoe is the downward slope created by the higher heel and lower forefoot. When the heel is higher than the forefoot, it encourages heel-striking, which may be why up to 80 percent of runners today land on their heels. Some overbuilt shoes are produced with the heel 12–15 millimeters higher than the forefoot, which creates up to a 17 percent downward slope angle. Shoes that are best for running naturally should have less than a 5-degree ramp angle.

Concerns of Safety and Environment

Even though the skin on the sole of your foot is tougher than skin on other parts of your body, running barefoot can expose your bare sole to splinters, cuts from rocks and glass shards, and bee stings (while running through clover, for example). Your bare, unprotected foot is also vulnerable to so-called thermal injury caused by temperature extremes of the running surface, leading to burns and freezing.

FACT

Although shoes provide protection from the elements and from hazardous surfaces, plenty of runners have run barefoot in training and competition and have performed well. Ethiopian runner Abebe Bikila ran barefoot and won the 1960 Olympics marathon. In the 1980s, Zola Budd-Pieterse of South Africa also ran barefoot competitively at the international level.

Energy Return

Current evidence suggests that the soft landing of the bare foot on the ground has inherent shock-absorbing characteristics. Running unshod also encourages a decreased stride length, the initial contact of the foot under the body's center of gravity, and the natural dampening of shock by the arch of the foot, ankle, knee, and hip. The design of your foot also allows it to store energy in the plantar fascia, muscles, and ligaments, and then uncoil and return this energy by the time your foot leaves the ground. No matter what the marketing hype proclaims, the modern cushioned running shoe returns only a small fraction of the absorbed energy that is returned by the structures of your unshod foot.

ALERT

Senior citizens beware: Barefoot running may be harder on less-resilient older feet. As we age, we adapt more slowly to physical change, we heal more slowly, and we lose flexibility and strength. This is not to say that the older runner cannot adapt to barefoot running, but that the transition may take longer and there may be some setbacks.

Medical Considerations

Some less-than-perfect foot characteristics may prevent you from running barefoot. Conditions such as *hypo*mobility (stiffness) or *hyper*mobility (floppiness) of the foot or imbalances in the forefoot sometimes need to be corrected by an orthotic or by some of that high-tech footwear.

Some medical conditions will also prevent individuals from participating in barefoot running. Those with osteoporosis or peripheral arterial disease should not run without shoes. A common complication for those with diabetes is the loss of protective sensation on their feet due to peripheral neuropathy. Walking or running barefoot is not recommended for those with sensation loss in their feet.

Retraining the Barefoot Way

To run barefoot, you will need to learn to run on the midfoot or forefoot. You should begin on a flat surface such as pavement, packed sand, or a dirt trail. Because your feet are unaccustomed to running without shoes, you will naturally run with a very light footstrike on your midfoot or forefoot. Without shoes on your feet, landing on your heels will feel uncomfortable and unnatural.

Run Lightly

Some experts endorse running on a soft surface such as grass in the beginning. Running on a soft surface has advantages and disadvantages. The less-compliant surface will force you to use more muscles in your feet and ankles to compensate for the irregularity of the ground. That's good. However, when running on a soft surface, you are less likely to land lightly on your foot, which you will need to do when you eventually transition to running on harder surfaces.

Be patient when beginning a barefoot running program and plan on it taking *months* for tissue adaptation to occur for muscles, tendons, and ligaments in the feet and ankles. The skin on the soles of your feet and the fat pad on your heel will also need to adapt to the abrasive surfaces you may encounter. You will need adequate strength and flexibility throughout your feet and lower legs. If you are overzealous and impatient, then you risk injuries such as Achilles tendinitis, plantar fasciitis, calf muscle strain, and a host of strains, sprains, and pains in your feet.

ALERT

It is very important to begin retraining the barefoot way when you are *healthy and injury-free*. From there, you follow a conditioning approach of progressive overload as you would for any exercise program. You begin by introducing short periods of alternating walking and running barefoot, then gradually increase the distance (or time) of the barefoot running to allow the body to adapt.

Shifting Your Load

When adopting the correct barefoot running form, it will be necessary for your foot to strike the ground below your center of mass; that is, beneath your knee, not ahead of it. Overstriding occurs when your step is too long and you land with your foot forward of your center of gravity. Overstriding is a common problem of heel-strikers. One way to reduce overstriding is to run at a faster cadence, say 170–180 steps per minute. You can use a metronome or some upbeat music of a suitable tempo to help you to find and maintain this optimal cadence. You will find it very hard to overstride at 170–180 steps per minute.

How It's Done

The actual mechanics of learning to run barefoot are simple. Warm up with a barefoot walk of 5–10 minutes, then start a stopwatch and begin jogging. Your steps should be short and you should land lightly on your midfoot—not on your heel. Opinions vary as to the best surface to start with. It might depend on how tough the soles of your feet are. If you have been walking around barefoot all summer before beginning your barefoot running, you would probably be comfortable running on a synthetic track or a smooth, hard surface such as a sidewalk. On the other hand, if your feet are soft and tender from years of shoes and socks, you may be better off beginning your barefoot running on short grass, packed sand, or a dirt path.

Although there is no scientifically proven best way to begin your program, experts agree that it is important to run barefoot not more than every other day for at least the first month. On the days that you are not running, you should be performing a set of exercises to strengthen your core, legs, and feet. Calf, hamstring, and foot flexibility are also important.

Exercises to Prepare You

Some exercises to strengthen the intrinsic muscles of your feet and the muscles of your ankles and lower leg include:

- **Marble pick-up:** While keeping your heel on the ground, rotate your foot inward and pick up a marble with your toes. Then move your foot outward and put down the marble. Repeat 20 to 30 times.
- **Tripod exercise:** Sit in a chair with your knee bent and your foot flat on the floor, press your big toe downward, and hold for 5 seconds. Repeat 10 to 20 times. Progress to performing the tripod exercise while standing, then while standing on one leg, and finally, by performing a lunge while pressing your big toe downward.
- **Tripod with body rotation:** Stand with feet shoulder-width apart. Perform simultaneous tripod big-toe press-downs while rotating your body first to the left and then to the right. Repeat 10 to 15 times.
- **Single leg tripod with body rotation:** Stand on one foot and perform a tripod big-toe push-down while rotating your body outward (you may need to hold onto something for balance). Perform 5 to 10 times on each leg.
- **Climbers:** Place your hands high up on a wall. Lift one knee high while rising up onto the toes of the opposite foot. Lower down and repeat 10 times for each leg.
- **Eccentric Achilles loading:** With your knees slightly bent, rise up onto the toes of both feet, lift one foot off the ground, and slowly lower the other heel to the ground. Perform 30 to 50 times on each leg.
- **Proprioception training:** Balance on one leg while standing on a 30- to 40-degree decline slant board (with your toe aiming down and a slight load off your heel).

Two Sample Progressions

Just as no two feet are alike, there is no single program to transition to barefoot running that is suitable for everyone. Here are two safe, comfortable options. Decide for yourself which of these running progressions suits you, or customize a plan that fits your experience and physical abilities. Some sources suggest that it may take up to a year to fully adapt to barefoot running.

Running Progression from Matthew Walsh, PT

The first four weeks of this program follows a run/walk format. The adaptation time may be longer for some runners who have poor biomechanics or who have worn highly cushioned shoes for most of their life.

Before you begin:

- Be able to walk (in shoes) at least 45 minutes every other day for two weeks
- Be comfortable doing some light double-legged jump roping for 2 minutes on the non-walking days

Begin the program sensibly as follows:

- **Week One:** Run barefoot for 1 minute followed by 4 minutes of barefoot walking. Repeat this run/walk ratio six or eight times every other day.
- **Week Two:** Run barefoot for 2 minutes followed by 3 minutes of barefoot walking. Repeat this run/walk ratio six or eight times every other day.
- **Week Three:** Run barefoot for 3 minutes followed by 2 minutes of barefoot walking. Repeat this run/walk ratio six or eight times every other day.
- **Week Four:** Run barefoot for 4 minutes followed by 1 minute of barefoot walking. Repeat this run/walk ratio six or eight times every other day. From here on, you can run continuously from 25–30 minutes every other day. Increase your distance or running time at a rate of 10 percent per week.

Vibram USA's Recommendations

This conservative approach highly recommends that you begin with a two-week program of re-education and strengthening before you start running (either barefoot or in minimalist shoes):

- **Weeks One and Two:** Perform the following exercises in three sets of 20 repetitions, three to five times per week:
  - ➤ Heel raises: Raise up and down on your toes
  - ➤ Dorsi-flexion/plantar-flexion: Slowly pump your feet up and down
  - ➤ Toe grip: Flex your toes and grip the floor with them
  - ➤ Toe spread/toe trap: Spread your toes apart, then press the big toe down to the floor (trap)
  - ➤ Exaggerated inversion and eversion: Slowly tip your feet so your soles face each other (inversion) then turn them so they face apart (eversion)
  - ➤ Grab a towel off the floor with your toes on one foot, then pass the towel to the toes of the other foot
  - ➤ Walk in your minimalist shoes for 1–2 hours a day
- **Weeks Three and Four:**
  - ➤ Warm up with the preceding foot exercises. Gently stretch your calves and arches.
  - ➤ Run 10 percent of your normal running distance no more than once every other day; for example, if your usual run is 3 miles, you should begin with running ¼ mile barefoot.
- **Weeks Five through Twelve:**
  - ➤ Warm up with the preceding foot exercises. Gently stretch your calves and arches.
  - ➤ Each week, increase your running distance by not more than 10 percent of the previous week's distance. Run every other day.
- **Weeks Thirteen and on:**
  - ➤ Warm up with the preceding foot exercises. Gently stretch your calves and arches.
  - ➤ Gradually increase the distance and frequency of your running, but listen to your body. Be patient while building your mileage slowly, and back off if you develop foot, ankle, or calf pain.

Injuries and Barefoot Running

Michael Warburton, PT, MSc, found in his review of research literature that although clinical research is lacking, there is a lower risk of lower leg injuries in the barefoot running population when compared to shod runners. He suggests that an increase in the number of injuries in modern running shoes is due to decreased sensory feedback provided from the foot and ankle. Foremost among these injuries are plantar fasciitis, shin splints, and iliotibial band friction syndrome.

Are Shoes Really Necessary?

It is believed that by running barefoot on firm surfaces, you naturally adjust your foot placement so that you land on your midfoot and thereby make a softer landing. This midfoot striking allows the arch of the foot to flex and absorb shock while allowing the musculature and support structures of the foot to control motion and lessen impact forces. This results in less damaging strain on tissue from your foot up to your lower back.

QUESTION

Are we destined to be injured?
Some experts believe that since very few runners are biomechanically perfect, most will need some sort of corrective or supportive shoes to prevent or reduce the risk of injury. Other experts say that the rate of running injuries is essentially unchanged since the introduction of the modern running shoe in the 1970s, and that some injuries, such as those involving the knee and Achilles tendon, may have increased in the past forty years.

Maybe the human foot was not meant to have a shoe that forces it to heelstrike, controls its pronation, blunts its sensory feedback, or provides cushion for its landing. Proponents of barefoot running believe that reliance on the external support, protection, and correction provided by the long-term use of footwear prevents the natural response of the well-functioning foot. Arch supports and orthotics added to the shoes may interfere even more by blocking the natural deflection of the arch. Granted, some of the less biomechanically gifted runners will need all of the things that the modern running shoe provides. Perhaps these runners are not well-suited for barefoot running. For others, less is better.

Give Yourself Time

Matthew Walsh, PT, advances the principle of "tissue adaptation time." When you remove the support of the running shoe, you place the control of motion for the foot and leg in the structures of the foot itself. Any tissue that operates at an extreme condition (shortened, lengthened, compressed, or torsioned) is less capable of controlling motion and adapting. This makes its adaptation time longer. During this time of tissue adaptation, secondary structures such as bone, cartilage, and tendon will be absorbing more load or stretch. Therefore, during this vulnerable period while you are transitioning to barefoot running, patience and time are necessary to prevent overload and breakdown of tissue.

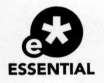

ESSENTIAL

Many symptoms that occur following an injury, such as pain and inflammation, are part of the body's adaptation process and should be expected.

Those runners blessed with good technique and mechanics will adapt easiest to barefoot running, while those with poor mechanics/alignment may have more trouble and need more time to transition to barefoot running. Practically speaking, if you possess the extremes of a high, rigid arch or a flat foot, you will likely need a longer time for tissues to adapt. The progressive loading and stress to this tissue needs to begin with short bouts of exposure that very gradually increase as they are spread out over a long period of time (weeks or months).

Consult an Expert

According to Vibram USA's Georgia Shaw, the majority of injuries associated with minimalist shoes and barefoot running in general are due to training errors and overuse. Keep in mind that by overloading tissue that is not accustomed or adapted to new demands, strain on bones and stress on connective tissue may lead to an increased risk of injuries such as stress fractures, plantar fasciitis, and tendonitis. If you are struggling with pain or are not able to progress with your barefoot running, you may need to consult a physical therapist or a physician who specializes in sports medicine for a thorough foot examination and assessment of your running mechanics.

Running Barefoot . . . in Shoes?

For some, the risk of foot injury due to puncture wounds, bruising, and thermal injury is not worth the benefit of running naturally and efficiently. This is where the minimalist shoe enters the picture. The minimalist shoe is light, flat, and snug. It allows you to feel the ground and to use your feet the way nature intended.

Shoe Makers Are Responding

According to Alan Rice, co-owner of Fleet Feet Sports, a running specialty store in Chico, California, even before Vibram began manufacturing their running lineup of shoes, other shoe manufacturers had begun developing lighter and lower profile training shoes. To respond to market demand, in addition to the shoes with ramp angles of 8 degrees, 10 degrees, and 12 degrees, shoe makers are manufacturing lines of 3-degree and 4-degree ramp angles and a thinner, more flexible sole. Today, New Balance, Saucony, Brooks, and others also market their own minimalist running shoes.

ESSENTIAL

If you plan to transition from typical running shoes to minimalist shoes, it is recommended that you first run barefoot until you develop your forefoot running form, then transition to the minimalist shoes. By running barefoot first, the tender skin of your feet will ensure that you do not push yourself too hard while you develop your forefoot running technique. Otherwise, there may be a tendency for the novice forefoot striker to overdo it without allowing ample time to develop the necessary lower leg and foot strength.

If you need to wear orthotics in your running shoes, running barefoot or in thin-soled shoes may not be for you. However, some orthotic wearers are able to transition from heel-striking to a forefoot running form and no longer need the support and control of an orthotic or an overbuilt running shoe.

The Minimalist Shoe

Minimalist shoes do not have a thick, cushioned heel like the typical running shoe, so, like barefoot running, your midfoot or forefoot will naturally strike the ground first followed gently by your heel. This soft landing is the body's natural way to absorb and distribute impact forces. Therefore, a heavy shoe is not necessary to provide a cushioned sole, motion control, or shock attenuation when the foot with a minimal shoe is adequate.

A valuable advantage of the Vibram FiveFingers® shoes is that they do not have a limited shelf life like the heavily cushioned running shoes of today. According to Georgia Shaw of Vibram USA, the rule of thumb to replace the modern cushy-foam running shoe every 300–400 miles does not exist for their minimalist footwear. Since these shoes have no cushion to pack down or harden over time, the shoes can presumably last for years—or as long as it takes to wear a hole in the sole. That would take a nice bite out of your annual shoe budget.

CHAPTER 10

ChiRunning

ChiRunning® is based on the holistic concepts of T'ai Chi, including a mind-body connection, core engagement, alignment, cadence, and a unique running form. When used in combination, these elements reduce running injuries and improve efficiency. ChiRunning is an alternative running technique that can be adopted by the novice or experienced runner. It replaces the heavy, cushioned running shoe with a minimalist shoe and a midfoot running technique. Danny Dreyer developed this running method, ingenious in its simplicity, which, when properly learned and applied, is to make running a more pleasurable activity. ChiRunning is an activity that builds a strong link between your mind and your body.

What Is ChiRunning?

T'ai Chi is a Chinese martial art, one practice in a group of techniques that are martial arts applied with internal power. The term *T'ai* translates roughly to "the ultimate," and *Chi* means "life force," or "life energy." T'ai Chi involves focusing the mind solely on the movements of the form, which is believed to bring about a state of mental calm and clarity. T'ai Chi training involves five elements that are comprised of response drills, self-defense techniques, the use of weapons, and solo hand routines, known as forms. While in popular culture the image of T'ai Chi is typified by exceedingly slow movement, many T'ai Chi styles have secondary forms of a faster pace. ChiRunning is one such secondary form.

FACT

This chapter presents an overview of the principles of ChiRunning®. Danny Dreyer is the creator and chief disseminator of the ChiRunning concept, philosophy, methods, and technique. His book, *ChiRunning: A Revolutionary Approach to Effortless, Injury-Free Running*, is the definitive work on the subject. The information outlined in this chapter is not meant to replace the detailed explanation in the *ChiRunning* book, or demonstration on the *ChiRunning* DVD, or the instruction in a *ChiRunning* clinic.

In their book, *ChiRunning: A Revolutionary Approach to Effortless, Injury-Free Running*, Danny Dreyer and Katherine Dreyer describe ChiRunning as more than just a running technique: It is a paradigm that combines a mindfulness approach with running. A strong connection is made between mind and body in ChiRunning. In fact, ChiRunning might even be more about Chi than it is about running. While you are running, your brain receives feedback information from all over your body, which it uses to control the intricate balance of the body lean (the body's leaning), posture, alignment, and armswing. Relaxation is also a key component of ChiRunning. Once again, it is your mind that allows you to relax. If all of this sounds mentally fatiguing to you, it should! In ChiRunning, the mind is *supposed* to be working harder than the body.

Thanks to its lower impact forces and a focus on running form and technique, ChiRunning may reduce your chances of becoming injured and allow you to run longer into your old age. Whereas standard running (non-ChiRunning) is goal-oriented or "results" oriented (to run faster, run farther, or achieve a goal of completing an event), ChiRunning focuses more on the *process* of running. ChiRunning makes running pleasurable by striving to make it physically effortless.

The philosophy and practice of ChiRunning and its application to other parts of your life goes well beyond the mechanics of running.

ChiRunning is comprised of several components. You can improve your running efficiency and technique by adopting any single component, but ChiRunning is the sum of the components all working together to move you over the ground. These components are a focused mind, a strong and engaged core, great posture, proper breathing technique, and relaxed limbs.

Three Key Principles Shared by T'ai Chi and ChiRunning

1. **"Needle in Cotton"**—This principle is built on the analogy of a needle, being formed by your core muscles holding your spine in proper alignment, which move in a ball of soft cotton representing your flexible and relaxed limbs. In ChiRunning, all movements of your body originate in your center. The chi center, in Eastern belief, is located just below the navel and in front of the spine. This is roughly the same location of our center of mass in the Western culture. As long as your center (the needle) is well aligned, your limbs will move freely around this center. In ChiRunning, you focus on moving your *center* forward, which takes the emphasis away from your legs propelling you. Efficient movement comes from the muscles of your core, not the leg muscles.

2. **Gradual Progress**—The principle of Gradual Progress states that all things must grow in an incremental process. This step-by-step growth applies not only to ChiRunning but to all development processes such as

physical skills, relationships, living organisms, and even ideas. A major factor in succeeding with the principle of gradual progress hinges on a valuable commodity: time. If you put in the time, and you are biomechanically sound, you can develop your long-distance running ability with ChiRunning.

3. **Balance in Motion**—In ChiRunning, the principle of Balance in Motion exists when complementary forces interact favorably with one another. This state of balance and centeredness is present when your alignment is optimal and you move forward. Your body lean is balanced with your stride opening behind you. The more you lean, the more your stride opens up. But if you lean too much, then muscle activity increases and efficiency declines. The key is to know where your center is and to find your balance point as you lean forward, then relax your limbs to avoid resistance that results in fatigue or injury.

Conventional thought is that the majority of running injuries are those of overtraining, also called "training errors." These are blunders that occur when you increase your weekly mileage too quickly or add hills or speed work to your training program before you are properly conditioned. Dreyer makes a strong argument for what he believes is the true cause of running injuries. He does not subscribe to the common belief that the primary cause of running injuries is overuse. Instead, he believes that running injuries are primarily caused by poor running form and poor biomechanics.

Form faults and biomechanical flaws cause undue stress on soft tissue, which will lead to the aches and pains of tissue breakdown. Whether the cause of running injuries is training errors or biomechanical inadequacies, they might be reduced or eliminated by adopting the ChiRunning form and by following the ChiRunning principle of Gradual Progress. With proper technique and a step-by-step progression, you can shorten your recovery time, reduce muscle soreness, and decrease running-related injuries.

The Elements of Chi (Running!)

ChiRunning is made up of many components. These components enhance both the mental and the physical aspects of your movement. Individually, these elements can improve your current running. When used together, they transform you into a ChiRunner!

Chi-Skills

Dreyer has laid out four Chi-Skills to be mastered by the ChiRunner. These skills can be carried over into your life to be used to reach your running and personal goals with greater ease. By practicing these Chi-Skills while you run, you will sharpen your ability to focus your mind, sense your body, relax, and maximize the benefits of breathing properly.

1. **Focusing Your Mind**—It is your mind that is doing most of the work while you are ChiRunning. It turns off the chatter in your brain and allows you to focus on the task at hand. It signals your muscles when to work and when to relax. Your mind is used to direct movements of the body to master a skill. Focusing Your Mind in ChiRunning trains your mind to sense, respond to, and direct movements of your body whether you are moving or still.

2. **Body Sensing**—Body Sensing is the most important of the four Chi-Skills. In order to improve your running technique, you need to develop the ability to sense when you are moving your body correctly and when you are moving it incorrectly. Body Sensing is the skill of having your mind and your body working together. When you are skilled at Body Sensing, you will be able to listen to the subtle messages from your body and immediately make the appropriate adjustments to your running form necessary to maintain your efficiency.

3. **Breathing**—Breathing is an important skill not only for the proper exchange of carbon dioxide for oxygen in your lungs but also for tying Relaxation and Body Sensing into ChiRunning. Many Eastern disciplines, including martial arts, meditation, and yoga, use breathing as a core component of their practice. The key is to breathe deeply to fill the bottom recesses of your lungs where most of the gas exchange takes place. Dreyer contends that shortness of breath while running is not occurring because you are not breathing *in* deeply enough, but because you are not *exhaling* enough air from the lower lungs. The most effective breathing method for drawing air into the lower lobes of your lungs is *diaphragmatic breathing*, also called "belly breathing."

4. **Relaxation**—The Chi-Skill of Relaxation is achieved by a combination of the first three Chi-Skills. If you are Focusing Your Mind, Body Sensing, and Breathing properly, then you can achieve relaxation with your running. Remember "Needle in Cotton" where your spine (represented by the needle) is held in proper upright alignment by your core muscles while at the same time your limbs (represented by the cotton) are relaxed and moving around your center.

So you can see that the mind really is more involved in ChiRunning than you may have thought. If you understand these four Chi-Skills, then you will understand what it really is to be ChiRunning. If you do not engage your mind, ChiRunning is little more than an alternative technique to improve running form and efficiency. By practicing these Chi-Skills in your everyday running, over time they will become second nature and you will find that they carry over into and enrich your everyday life.

Aligning Yourself

The key here is to create your "column." Your "column" is formed by proper alignment of the shoulders, hips, and ankles. When you find this optimal alignment, your skeleton will support you and your muscles can relax.

Danny Dreyer uses a connect-the-dots activity in the *ChiRunning* book and at the ChiRunning workshops to check your alignment and core strength. Have a partner stand behind you and press firmly downward on your shoulders. If your core is engaged and your column is properly aligned, you will be able to absorb the downward pressure without moving. If, on the other hand, you buckle somewhere in your column, your alignment needs to be improved. This activity is also used by some physical therapists to check your posture and alignment and is termed the vertical compression test. A physical therapist or a certified ChiRunning instructor can use this tool to teach you how to correct your alignment and stand properly.

Lean

In the traditional running stride, you reach out your foot by flexing your hip while pushing off from the opposite foot. But in ChiRunning, you use the lean of your body and the pull of gravity to power you. The technique involves leaning with your whole body *from the ankles* (like a Nordic ski jumper). Now catch yourself with your feet as you move forward. Not very much lean is necessary for this "gravity assist" to carry you forward. Dreyer describes a "window of lean" in which you are balanced—not too far forward, but not too upright either. Using gravity in this way reduces the workload on your muscles, reducing fatigue and improving efficiency.

Striding and Landing

In ChiRunning, you will keep your stride length short. It may seem counterintuitive to run with a short step, but it is actually more efficient than taking long ones. Your midfoot impacts the ground softly. As you move forward, lift your feet behind you and let the ground pass beneath you. Concentrate on moving your center and letting your relaxed arms and legs follow.

While ChiRunning, you will always run with a midfoot strike by landing with your foot beneath your center of mass. You do not reach out with your feet; instead, you use gravity to pull yourself forward, and you catch your fall with your midfoot strike. You will land in the midfoot section of your foot either directly under your knee or behind it. Your stride will open up behind you as you run faster.

It's All about Rhythm

Another fundamental feature of ChiRunning is maintaining a constant cadence no matter what pace you are running. Dreyer found the optimal cadence for energy efficiency and to prevent overstriding to be 170–180 steps (85–90 strides) per minute. When you speed up, your cadence stays the same and you lengthen your stride.

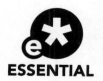

ESSENTIAL

Your cadence is measured as the number of *steps* you take in a minute. Since 170–180 steps are a lot to count, it is easier to measure the cadence in *strides* per minute. A stride is made up of two steps. So a stride rate of 85–90 means that your right foot will strike the ground 85–90 times per minute.

It takes practice to keep your legs moving at the same turnover rate while running at various speeds. Long, loping strides and high turnover are the two extremes of inefficient running. If you are taller and have longer legs, then you may be running closer to the 170 steps per minute, and if your legs are shorter you would target 180 steps per minute for your cadence.

Shifting Gears

Dreyer describes ChiRunning as having four gears to run various speeds while at the same time conserving energy. You use a shorter stride (1st gear) at the start and at lower speeds. You can easily shift gears by adding an inch at a time to your forward lean. Remember that ChiRunning is performed at a constant cadence, so as you lean forward at the ankles to engage higher gears, your legs will still be turning over at the same rate of 170–180 steps per minute, but your body will move over the ground faster and your stride will lengthen behind you.

- **1st gear:** This is a very slow, easy, and relaxed pace that is engaged by leaning just enough to get you moving forward. This is your warm-up speed.
- **2nd gear:** This medium speed is the speed at which you would do an average training run. It is a comfortable aerobic pace.
- **3rd gear:** This is the speed you would sustain during a race or performance event. This pace is at the high end of your aerobic capacity.
- **4th gear:** This is the sprint. It is an anaerobic pace that is used for shorter distances.

Pelvic Rotation

Since your cadence will be constant across the variety of speeds you run, it is your stride length behind you that changes as you speed up and slow down. A natural rotation point in your spine exists in the center of your body where the thoracic portion of your spine joins with your lower back (vertebrae T12/L1). When you engage your core and level your pelvis, your legs become an extension of your pelvis and are relaxed as your pelvis rotates. Remember, in ChiRunning your legs provide support from the ground, but are *not* powering your forward movement.

If your core is not engaged, then the connection between your pelvis and legs will be lost and you will be pushing from your legs instead of using gravity-assisted movement from your center. When shifting gears to speed up, it will be necessary for you to increase your pelvic rotation in order for your hip extension to increase as your stride opens behind you.

FACT

Bend your elbows at a 90-degree angle and swing them back from your shoulders. By swinging your elbows to the rear, you create a counter-balance to your forward lean. Keep your arms and hands relaxed with your wrists moving at the level of your waistband.

Using Your Y'chi

Dreyer explains *Y'chi* as the act of using your mind to direct the energy and movement of your body *through your eyes*. To use the Y'chi (pronounced "ee-chee") technique, focus on a distant object in front of you. Lock your eyes on the object and draw yourself toward it as you run. Try this visualization: pretend that a bungee cord is attached between your sternum and the object in the distance. Let the bungee cord gently pull you toward the object.

Getting Psyched

ChiRunning is not as much an activity as it is a practice. Building the physical skills is only part of it (Dreyer says this is 10 percent of ChiRunning). There is much more mental activity involved than simply putting in your miles and doing your drills. It is a practice of mastering the ability to listen to your body, optimize your breathing, and balance your forward movement with your stride. ChiRunning is a mindful activity like meditation is a mindful activity. Done properly, over time, it will improve your quality of running and your quality of living. ChiRunning is also about letting go of tension in your life—not only physical tension, but emotional tension and stress.

Making the Adjustments

ChiRunning is a practice. There are many elements for you to perfect over time. Each time you go out you can focus on a different aspect of the Chi-Running technique. Think about your posture, your core, your armswing, your cadence, your breathing. . . .

Feeling the Chi

Hazel Wood, certified ChiRunning instructor, explains that it takes time to "feel" within your body. Appreciate what it *feels* like to feel the ground under your feet, the subtle lean of your body, and the movement of your armswing. Some elements of the ChiRunning technique might come very easy to you. Maybe it's the feeling of the balance between your gravity-assisted lean and your back-kick. Or maybe it's your cadence or your arm-swing. Wood recommends focusing during the early stages of learning on those elements that come naturally and easily to you rather than working hard on the elements that are effortful.

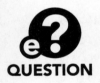

QUESTION

How long will it take to learn ChiRunning?
To fully adopt the ChiRunning technique takes most people about three months. Dreyer states that most people feel 95 percent better while running by the end of a ChiRunning workshop.

If you currently run in one of those heavy, cushioned, high-heeled running shoes, Dreyer recommends a progression to a lighter, flatter shoe for ChiRunning. A safe progression can be accomplished in one of two ways: (1) drop your running mileage and go straight into a minimal-ist shoe, or (2) you can continue with your current mileage but change from the heavy shoe first to a neutral trainer, then to a racing flat. Either way, you must apply the principle of Gradual Progress while making the transition.

The ChiRunning Movement

Dreyer describes the ChiRunning movement as one of growth worldwide. His book, which is *a must* for anyone serious about learning ChiRunning, first printed in 2004, is printed in ten languages at this writing. There are at least 145 certified ChiRunning instructors in twenty countries and almost 200,000 runners have attended ChiRunning workshops.

FACT

ChiWalking was born in 2008 out of popular demand and is based on the fundamentals of ChiRunning.

Momentum for the ChiRunning movement is gathering as more people become interested in running in minimalist shoes.

The Best Way to Learn It

The *ChiRunning* book and an associated DVD are available at the ChiRunning website (*www.chirunning.com*). If you want to learn the ChiRunning technique, you can take a ChiRunning workshop (they are offered all over the world). Although you can understand and practice the elements of the ChiRunning technique, there is no substitute for having a certified ChiRunning instructor teach you and critique your form. Dreyer estimates that the biomechanics of ChiRunning is only about 10 percent of what it is to be a ChiRunner.

Hazel Wood, certified ChiRunning instructor, states that the most common form error she observes in fledgling ChiRunners is leaning too much. The proper forward lean is much less than most people think. Without instruction, people will often heel-strike and take too long a stride. They will also tend toward not relaxing their legs enough, which leads to underutilizing the effect of gravity and overusing their legs.

Danny and Katherine Dreyer clearly and expertly lay out ChiRunning drills called Form Focuses in their *ChiRunning* book. Form Focuses clearly explain the posture, alignment, and core strengthening techniques needed for ChiRunning. The Dreyers have also created a three-disk audio series (also available in an MP3 format) that talks a runner through the ChiRunning form.

Alternative Applications

ChiRunning techniques are being applied to treating runners undergoing physical therapy. Concepts such as alignment and core strength are common to both ChiRunning and techniques applied by Certified Functional Manual Therapist (CFMT) physical therapists trained through the Institute of Physical Art.

Physical Therapy and ChiRunning

Proper spinal alignment and control of posture are central elements to ChiRunning. If a runner is unable to simulate or sustain the ChiRunning position, physical therapy techniques can be applied to address the runner's particular problem. According to Noelle Righter-Freer, PT, MPT, CFMT, sources of running injuries can be categorized in three ways: structural deficits, neuromuscular deficits, and motor control deficits. Hands-on techniques are used to address the structural and neuromuscular deficits, whereas some therapists, such as Righter-Freer and others, are using ChiRunning techniques as an adjunct to treating the motor control deficits.

After any structural or neuromuscular deficits are corrected, optimal alignment of your column can be evaluated using the vertical compression test (described earlier). The physical therapist teaches you to correct your alignment in order to eliminate any buckling or shear on your joints. Once you understand how to properly align your column while standing upright, the same alignment must be maintained when you are in the gravity-assisted position of leaning forward from your ankles while ChiRunning or ChiWalking.

ChiRunning Versus Barefoot Running

ChiRunning goes hand in hand with minimalist shoes running. Minimalist shoes running goes hand in hand with barefoot running. In some ways

ChiRunning and barefoot running are compatible, but in other ways they are not.

The Similarities

From a purely mechanical standpoint, both barefoot running and Chi-Running techniques employ a slight forward lean and the same higher cadence of 170–180 steps per minute. They also both avoid overstriding by using a shorter step with the foot landing beneath the knee and by not striking with the heel. In both techniques you lift your foot and avoid using your legs for propulsion by pushing off. Both require that you run relaxed. Both employ the strategy of "gradual progress" and have an adaptation period in which you slowly build your tolerance and technique with practice over a period of time. ChiRunning is indeed a "barefoot-like" running form you can use whether you're wearing shoes or not.

The Differences

With barefoot running the posture is more erect and there is less emphasis on core strength. Although neither technique involves heel-striking, Chi-Running technique uses a midfoot strike, whereby the purists in barefoot running contact the ground more with their forefoot.

Perhaps the most striking difference between barefoot running and ChiRunning is the mind-body connection. Whereas barefoot running gives you the feel and freedom of natural running, ChiRunning goes beyond the purely physical mechanics of form and incorporates a mind-body approach that barefoot running tends to lack. Barefoot running can be used to supplement your running regimen, whereas ChiRunning is a form change that you adopt, learn, and apply.

Dreyer describes ChiRunning as having a "barefoot-like" feel. Some people can ChiRun completely unshod, but would probably be limited on the surfaces they can run on and the steepness of the downhill grade they are comfortable with. ChiRunning can potentially replace your old heel-striking, heavily shod, overstriding running form with an efficient running technique and mindful centeredness.

CHAPTER 11

Alternative Techniques for Mental and Physical Strength

Runners of all abilities have discovered the many benefits of cross-training as a means to enhance total conditioning and running performance. They have also found that sharpening their mental state and learning to connect to their bodies helps overall running performance as well. Yet despite the variety and popularity of cross-training options, some runners still question why they should incorporate activities from cycling to yoga into their training programs if running is their primary focus.

Pilates

The Pilates fitness system was originally called "Contrology" by its founder, Joseph Pilates. Of German and Greek descent, Joseph Pilates emigrated to the United States in 1926 and opened a studio in New York City where he and his wife, Clara, taught his particular exercise method. Pilates' concept was to focus on core postural muscles to support the spine for correct alignment, an approach adopted by hospital rehabilitation programs ever since. Used for years as the exercise routine of choice by professional dancers, recently the Pilates system has become very popular with the general public, particularly with those looking for a gentle method of increasing core strength, flexibility, and movement.

Pilates is typically taught in health clubs, where private or semiprivate instruction is available on specialized Pilates equipment or group mat classes are conducted without equipment. Pilates uses resistance provided by the body to condition and correct itself, with the goal of lengthening and aligning the spine. Like yoga, Pilates offers a low-impact form of strengthening and toning muscles while helping you get more in tune with your body.

Yoga

If you have not yet at least taken a yoga class by now, what are you waiting for? Yoga classes and studios continue to pop up everywhere these days, making it convenient and easy to explore this ancient tradition of body, mind, and spirit. Yoga instructor Suzanne Goldston explains:

The intimate interplay between the body and the mind is the essence of yoga. Creating balance in the body without creating balance in the mind will bring only limited success. If mind and body cooperate then physical balance can be achieved by locating imbalances and adjusting them. Balance requires precise attention. You could say yoga is similar to walking a tightrope: you are never stationary, but always adjusting to the movement of the rope.

Increasingly, runners are finding that yoga, in contrast to more strenuous forms of cross-training, provides them with additional strength and flexibility without beating up their joints. Bearing in mind that skeletal muscles work in pairs, what happens during running is that the foot, leg, and hip muscles experience a heavy amount of pounding, tightening, and shortening. Left unattended, these compromised muscles are stressed, possibly leading to injury. Stretching brings them back into balance, keeping them soft and supple so they can do their job.

ALERT

Since muscles help maintain posture and balance, if these are out of sync, the stressful demands of running will aggravate any pre-existing conditions. Many runners simply run in pain and learn to live with it. Yoga can help identify and treat these nagging sources of pain, leading to more enjoyable running—and more years of it.

As an athlete, you can benefit from yoga in at least three major ways: (1) Since yoga both stretches and strengthens the body, it promotes physical balance; (2) mental alertness is increased; and (3) injuries and discomforts are more easily prevented with a consistent yoga practice. Certainly we have felt refreshed and attentive after exercise. This is due to the fact that the activity has stimulated the action of the muscles in pumping fluids through the body.

More efficient pumping by muscles depends on their level of elasticity. Such elasticity will increase through the practice of yoga. In the same way, increased muscular flexibility and strength will prevent many common injuries and annoyances, such as muscle pulls and stiffness, associated with strenuous exercise.

The power for athletic movement is the result of contraction, or shortening, of muscles. Stretching can counteract the negative effects of repeated contractions that occur during running and other sports. All athletic exertion can be viewed as repetitive and coordinated contraction of muscles and muscle groups. The resting length of the muscle *spindle*, the message center of the muscle, is determined by such continual contractions. When the spindle learns that the muscles are being asked to continually shorten, it adjusts to the demands and becomes increasingly resistant to stretching or lengthening. Muscles that are persistently worked without stretching can thus become hard and short. Stiff muscles deprive the body by inhibiting the movement of joints, prohibiting full contraction of the opposing muscles, misaligning the body, decreasing body efficiency, increasing the possibility of injury, and deterring the maximum pumping action within each muscle.

Ballistic stretching is a forced, jerky process used by some runners to try to force muscle toward a certain position beyond its normal range. The completed stretch is seldom held more than a few seconds, with the intention of achieving a predetermined degree of flexibility. This method of stretching is an attempt by the mind to force the body into an idealized form. The brain is trying to dictate to the body with little or no dialogue between body and mind, with only the most intense bodily feelings being heeded by the brain.

By contrast, yoga stretching uses a slow, steady motion to enter a pose, the person gently holding at the limit of his or her stretch for 10 seconds to 10 minutes or longer. This slower, less forceful approach gives you greater control over the positioning, safety, and efficiency of each pose as well as allowing you to look and feel within to see how the body and mind are responding to the poses. The precision necessary for each pose guides you to physical balance.

In yoga, "success" is measured by your inward attention to the body and mind. No matter how flexible you are, you will benefit from yoga. It is simply a matter of being willing to feel and respond to yourself.

Finding Your Style

Trace Bonner, Director of Holy Cow Yoga Center in Charleston, South Carolina, explains:

When Yoga emerged in the United States around the turn of the 20th century it was an obscure practice from India and consisted of various approaches. The most commonly known types of yogas that are still practiced in India include Karma Yoga (service), Jnana Yoga (reflective), Bhakti Yoga (devotional), and Raja Yoga (meditation). The most popular approach in the United States, however, is Hatha Yoga, meaning to balance the body through physical postures (asanas), breathing exercises (pranayama), and relaxation (yoga nidra). Throughout this past century, many Hatha Yoga teachers in India and the United States gained prominence through their varying styles, which have emerged, expanded, and overlapped into an intricate web of yoga teachers and practices.

Bonner further explains that there are several yoga styles available to study and practice. The following is a list of just some of today's styles for the individual to choose from:

FROM INDIA

- **Iyengar Yoga®:** Anytime you walk into a studio that has a block, strap, pillow, or bolster, we can thank B. K. S. Iyengar. While some Iyengar® studios are purist, meaning they stick strictly to Iyengar's sequence and alignment principles, others are influenced by his use of props to help students find a proper alignment and support throughout the practice. You will like this style if you like precision.
- **Ashtanga Yoga:** We can thank Sri K. Pattabhi Jois for any yoga class that moves with fluidity, such as Vinyasa style. Jois's teachings come directly from Krishnamacharya (1888–1989), an established yoga master, healer, and scholar. Jois delineated Primary Series, a series of seventy-two postures done with vinyasa (linking breath and movement), drishti (eye focus), and ujjayi breath ("victorious breath"). You will like this style if you like strength and structure.
- **Bikram Yoga®:** This practice is hot—really hot! Heating the room to 105 degrees, this class, sequenced by Bikram Choudhury, consists of twenty-six postures meant for cleansing the body. You will like this style if you like it hot and sweaty.
- **Sivananda® Yoga:** Arising from the influence of yoga as a practice for healing the body, Swami Sivananda created an inclusive sequence of breathing, postures, relaxation, and meditation. Sivananda wrote around 200 books during his life on yoga and its healing effects for body and mind. You will like this style if you like a well-rounded and simplistic inward practice.

- **Jivamukti Yoga®:** Creators Shannon Gannon and David Life, after many years of practice with K. Pattabhi Jois, take the principles of Ashtanga but infuse it with their own fluidity and social activisim. Each class begins with a dharma talk (spiritual teaching), chanting (spiritual song), then a rousing and sweaty posture sequence along with strong adjustments, and followed by relaxation. You will like this style if you like learning how to be a better person on and off the mat.
- **Anusara® Yoga:** Gaining prominence in recent years, creator John Friend brings principles of alignment and heart to the practice. Each posture is about opening to grace and joy. You will like this style if you like joyful expression.
- **Baptiste Power Vinyasa Yoga®:** With a more intense, Western-centric style of yoga, Baron Baptiste never lets the practice wane as you rocket through postures in his carefully sequenced series of Baptiste Power Vinyasa Yoga®. Baron comes from a family yoga lineage, and he continues that through his own unique style. You will like this style if you like it fast and rigorous.
- **OM Yoga:** Rising into her own right, OM Yoga creator Cyndi Lee infuses the practice with her own eclectic style of Ashtanga and Iyengar Yoga® and Buddhist teachings, as well as a generous sense of humor. You will like this style if you like a fluid, playful, and yet meditative practice.

There are many more styles, such as Kundalini, Integral®, Viniyoga™, Phoenix Rising Yoga Therapy, Ananda, Himalayan Institute, to name just a few. And, when determining which Hatha Yoga style is right for you, you must be willing to explore the ever-expanding plethora of teachers and yoga studios.

Turning the Focus Inward

Yoga focuses the mind on the internal movements of the body so that mind, body, and breath are integrated. In a 2002 article in *Yoga Journal* on how yoga and running complement each other, Baron Baptiste and Kathleen Finn Mendola write:

In addition to physically counteracting the strains of running, yoga teaches the cultivation of body wisdom and confidence. As you develop a greater understanding of the body and how it works, you become able to listen and respond to messages the body sends you. This is especially important in running, where the body produces a lot of endorphins. These "feel good" chemicals also double as Nature's painkillers, which can mask pain and the onset of injury or illness. Without developed body intuition, it's easier to ignore the body's signals.

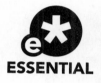

ESSENTIAL

International spiritual leader, artist, and activist Sri Chinmoy said: "The body's capacity and the soul's capacity, the body's speed and the soul's speed, go together. Running and physical fitness help us both in our inner life of aspiration and in our outer life of activity." Check out the aspirations and accomplishments of the Sri Chinmoy Marathon Team at *www.srichinmoyraces.org*.

Other Benefits

Yoga's focus on breathing can be extremely beneficial to runners. In fact, the *Indian Journal of Medical Research* published a study showing that athletes who practiced yogic breathing (pranayama) were able to exercise more intensely at the same heart rate compared to those who didn't. According to the Pranayama Institute in New Mexico, "The system of pranayama is credited with conferring upon its practitioner a calm, balanced, and focused mind, increased vitality, and longevity."

Meditation

"Just a minute," you might be saying. "How does sitting and thinking about nothing benefit my running program?" Trace Bonner, director of Holy Cow Yoga Center in Charleston, South Carolina, explains:

Loosely translated, meditation means bring to the center, specifically the mind. When we allow the mind to find a centered space it feels relaxed and easeful. The way we get the mind to center is usually not easy, due to the fact that the mind is always thinking and commenting through an inner dialogue. This pulls the mind out of center and into personal perception, judging, comparing and identification. In order to bring the mind to center, a technique is used, such as concentration on the breath, uplifting word, mantra, walking . . . and running (just to name a few).

Meditative Running

Meditation can also be practiced while you are running. As one runs, and becomes aware of each step the foot makes to the pavement—concentrating on where the foot is stepping, the breath during the run, the response of the body as it runs—your mind can become focused and thereby centered. As the mind stays centered, you might begin to feel less tied to the stress in life as well as to your relationship to that stress. In other words, you might feel less emotionally tied to the effects of stress. This is the benefit of meditation. The mind steps into center and we have an opportunity to release the attachments of the way we think about our lives.

Meditation can be likened to *the zone* that many people have felt when doing something with steady concentration. As the mind becomes fully engaged in a single activity, we move out of thinking and into experiencing. The right brain activity increases, time slows down, and we drop into *being* in the moment. Because we are usually dominant in left-brain activity, which perceives, judges, compares, and identifies, the balance of engaging the right brain brings the mind into a balanced and centered state. This has enormous benefits for physical and mental health, as well as our spiritual development.

While running can be meditative, it might be good to explore the traditional seated meditation experience. For as much as active meditations can be beneficial, the deeper benefits of the practice can be felt when the body is still. For it is said that when the body is still then the mind becomes steady and still. While the mind can never stop thinking (that's its job), we can create pauses between the thoughts, whereby less thinking is taking place. In the pauses, which can be extended and expanded, a tremendous awareness of peace can be found, and a deeper connection to spirit experienced.

Benefits of meditation include:

- Increased blood flow
- Increased brainwave coherence
- Increased self-confidence and feelings of well-being
- Increased exercise tolerance
- Decreased muscle tension
- Decreased blood pressure
- Decreased anxiety, depression, and moodiness

Do some research, and you'll soon discover that meditation can benefit you physically, psychologically, and spiritually. And a better you makes a better runner.

Reiki

Reiki is a spiritual healing art, one that uses a natural system of touch healing. Hands-on healing has been practiced for centuries, but the unique form of energy healing called Reiki was started by a Japanese man named Mikao Usui in March 1922. Since then millions of people from all around the world have learned about Reiki's benefits as a complementary and alternative medicine (CAM).

World-renowned cardiothoracic surgeon, author, and TV host Dr. Mehmet Oz fully endorses Reiki; his wife is a practitioner, and Reiki masters work alongside him during his open-heart surgeries and afterward in the recovery room to aid with faster healing time. Dr. Oz has seen firsthand that Reiki can help to release physical pain, remove energy obstructions, and help people destress from the daily grind.

According to holistic healer and certified life coach Avalaura Beharry, Reiki "is a simple and effective form of hands-on healing that uses Universal Life Energy to help dissolve problems in the body, mind, and spirit. It is a natural approach to healing that is safe, gentle and non-invasive."

Carrie Kenady is a certified Reiki practitioner who owns Mount Pleasant Reiki just outside of Charleston, South Carolina. She has given Reiki to several clients who are devoted runners. She explains the benefits of Reiki to runners through a personal experience:

My father, who is a surgical oncologist and avid marathon runner, loves receiving Reiki treatments when he comes to visit. He was skeptical at first since he has been trained in Western medicine, but after one Reiki session the pain from his shin splints was drastically decreased. He now believes that runners like himself can greatly benefit from Reiki and have less pain from pulled hamstrings, stress fractures, sprained ankles and other common runners' ailments.

In addition to physical healing, Reiki also provides spiritual and psychological benefits to runners. It aids with stress relief, tension, emotional discord, and anxiety. It is a soothing and deeply relaxing experience that provides peace and comfort. It cleanses and clears negative emotions and balances your energy. In essence, Reiki can do wonders for your pre-race jitters as well as your post-race physical ailments.

Consider Reiki as an alternative treatment as you progress in running. For more information on Reiki, visit *www.reiki.org*.

CHAPTER 12

Injury Prevention

Most running injuries are the result of training errors. To avoid injury, your increases in mileage and intensity should be gradual. It is important to vary hard days and easy days as well as hard and easy weeks. As a rule of thumb, you should increase mileage approximately 10 percent per week, and every fourth week you should back off on your mileage to allow your body to rest.

Avoiding Injury: The Basics

Most runners should devote at least one or two days a week to rest or non-running activities. This gives your body a chance to recover, rebuild, and heal itself. It is also helpful to maintain a running diary, which should contain your mileage, intensity, course, and brief notes on how you felt during each run. Such a record can help trace the origin of any number of training errors.

Not only do your mileage, frequency of running, the course you run, and the times you post matter, but there are other factors that contribute to how you feel and how your training progresses. You will find that taking note of physical infirmities like a scratchy throat, headache, or a bloated feeling can help you pinpoint when you began developing something more serious.

ESSENTIAL

The quality of your running can be affected by the medications you take, the amount you sleep at night, time changes when you travel, dietary changes, and increased stress on the job or at home. Your running diary may become so much more to you than a simple record, leaving you amazed when you look back after a year has gone by.

Treating Inflammation

Inflammation (characterized by pain, swelling, redness, and warmth) is an expected by-product of injury. When inflammation occurs at the site of an injury, treat the area with ice (see icing guidelines below). Above all, *do not* treat the area of an acute injury with heat of any kind, wet or dry, for several days.

Consider taking several days off from running and from any other sports that cause stress to an injured area. After 72 hours or so, you can try taking some anti-inflammatory medication (such as ibuprofen or naproxen sodium) for the injury, being careful to follow dosing instructions to ensure you maintain a therapeutic dose in your system. If the pain persists, see a physician for a thorough examination of the injury.

As long as the injury does not warrant immediate medical attention, icing can be the single most effective treatment for an acute injury. Apply ice to the area for 20 minutes and repeat this three to five times a day until the pain is gone. You can apply crushed ice, a cold pack, or a bag of frozen peas to do the icing. Do not ice for more than 20 minutes of each hour, because it *is* possible to develop frostbite if the tissue is very cold for too long.

Heat is a relaxing therapeutic measure that can be introduced later, after significantly reducing or eliminating inflammation of the injury site. Applying a hot pack wrapped in a towel for 10–15 minutes at a time may bring relief to minor injuries on the mend. But be sure to not overdo it, since heat is not an anti-inflammatory and it can cause swelling.

If all of these remedies fail, consider visiting a physician familiar with sports injuries and with experience treating runners to obtain an assessment of the injury and treatment advice. (Details on how to find a sports physician are found at the end of this chapter.) The most important information a physician can provide is whether you can continue to run without modification of your training schedule; if you can continue to run with a reduced workload; or if you must completely rest the injury site (that is, no running). Your physician can also tell you whether you should add cross-training activities to your schedule, both to maintain cardiovascular fitness and to strengthen the injury site.

FACT

To properly ice an injury, use an ice cup. Fill a small Styrofoam® cup with water and then place it in the freezer. When it is completely frozen, peel the top of the cup down to expose an inch or two of ice. Massage the injured area with the ice cup for 5–6 minutes until the area is numb. As the ice melts, peel down more of the cup and continue until the time is up. Ice the area again an hour or two later, but not more often than once per hour.

The Impact (Literally!) of Athletic Shoes

Running shoes should be replaced regularly to reduce your chances of injury. Many biomechanical problems can be corrected and running injuries prevented by the right pair of shoes. In fact, physical therapists and sports medicine physicians will look to the shoe for the source of running injuries from the knee down. The shock-absorbing capability of the shoe's midsole diminishes gradually and becomes inadequate after 350–500 miles. The number of miles depends on such factors as your weight, the training terrain, environmental conditions, and how light or heavy you are on your feet. Even if the upper part of the shoe does not show much wear, the shock-absorption quality may already be gone. If you are running approximately 20 miles per week, you should be replacing your shoes every 4–6 months, depending upon your shock-absorption needs. Use your runner's diary to note the condition of your running shoes. If you decide to change brands for any reason, you can track your comments as well as compare shoe performance.

Even if you are a careful runner, stretching consistently and not overextending yourself in your runs, you can incur injury from running in poorly designed shoes. By recognizing potential problems associated with faulty shoe design, you become a more discerning shoe buyer and ensure that the shoes you are wearing meet your biomechanical needs.

Shoes and Achilles Tendonitis

Shoes with inflexible soles cause the calf muscles to work harder and can contribute to the development of Achilles tendonitis, in which the Achilles tendon becomes inflamed. The mechanical reason for this is best explained by looking at the foot as a fulcrum-and-lever system. Shoes with inflexible soles make the lever arm (the foot) function over a longer distance and make the tip of the shoe the location of the fulcrum (the pivot point). Ideally, the shoe should flex at the point where the toes join the foot (which also happens to be the widest part of the shoe), offering more support. The shoes should also have a slight heel lift, which most running shoes do.

Shoes that have too much heel cushioning, including some air-cushioned models, can also contribute to Achilles tendonitis. After the heel strikes the ground, it continues moving as the shoe's cushioning continues to absorb shock. This continued motion can stretch a susceptible Achilles tendon excessively.

Shoes and Plantar Fasciitis

Running shoes that are too flexible in the midsole or that flex before the point at which the toes join the foot can both stretch the plantar fascia (the bowstring-like tissue on the sole of your foot) and contribute to excessive pronation in the foot. The resulting lack of stability occurs not just in the shoe's transverse plane (where the shoe actually flexes) but also in its longitudinal plane, thereby reducing the effectiveness of the shoe in controlling pronation.

FACT

Make sure you lace your shoes carefully before running. Too tight a shoe can make the tendons on the top of your foot sore or squeeze your *metatarsals* (long bones in the feet) too tightly. This in turn can result in feelings of numbness and/or tingling in your feet, particularly on long training runs. Too loose a shoe can make your foot less stable, resulting in excessive pronation and increasing the possibility of blisters.

Tips for Buying and Wearing Shoes

A shoe's midsole degrades from use. Given the lifespan of a running shoe, if you are running about 20 miles a week, you should consider changing shoes at weeks 20–25. Although the shoes are no longer good for running, they can still serve as casual wear for walking and for working in the yard. You can extend the life of your shoes somewhat by rotating back and forth between two pairs, so one same pair of shoes is not getting all the wear every time you run.

When assessing the condition of your running shoes, realize that even a new-looking shoe might lack adequate shock absorption. Use the 350- to 500-mile guideline instead of trying to guess how worn your shoes should look. Some runners mark the date they begin wearing the shoes in permanent marker somewhere on the shoe so they at least know how old the shoes are. You may want to track the mileage on your running shoes in your running log, too.

When buying your running shoes, make sure there is about a thumb's width between your toe and the front of the shoe. This helps prevent runner's (black) toe and/or losing your toenails. The shape and depth of the front of the shoe also affects these problems. When purchasing minimalist shoes, fit the shoe to your longest toe (which may not be your big toe).

Shoes have a shelf life. They lose about 100 miles of life per year in the closet even if they are never worn. For this reason, be careful of buying discount running shoes online. They may be selling "old" shoes that come to you with a reduced lifespan. Also, be wary of "running" shoes that are sold at department stores and retailers for $29.99, $39.99, and $49.99. Even if they are made by a major running shoe company, these sneakers are not real running shoes. Your best bet is to visit your local running shoe store and be fitted with a proper pair of running shoes. Plan on spending at least $100.

FACT

Don't even dream of running a marathon in a new pair of shoes. Your shoes should have at least 70 miles logged on them (including one long training run of 20 miles or longer) to be broken in well enough to run a marathon.

Guide to Shoes and Foot-Related Problems

The following list indicates appropriate shoe designs for certain foot conditions:

- **Low arch:** This condition may need support if you are an overpronator, so choose a stable shoe with good rear foot control.
- **High arch:** This foot may need more shock-absorption qualities in a shoe.
- **Normal foot:** This foot is ideal. You can avoid motion-control shoes and heavier shoes. This is a good foot for minimalist shoes.
- **Post-stress fracture:** Plan on replacing your shoes frequently (perhaps sooner than every 350–500 miles). Buy shoes with adequate shock absorption. You may need to make changes to your running form, training, or running surface as well.
- **Achilles tendonitis:** Tendonitis necessitates avoiding air soles, excessively spongy heels, and stiff-soled shoes.

Stretching to Prevent Injuries

As previously discussed, stretching cannot be emphasized enough as an injury-preventive routine. Runners frequently develop tightness in the posterior (those on the back side) muscle groups, which include the hamstrings and calf muscles. These same muscles can become relatively weak, which leads to an imbalance between the muscles in the front and those on the backs of your legs. The abdominal muscles also tend to be weak on runners who do not purposely strengthen them.

The Magic Six, Plus Two

The late George Sheehan, MD, recommended a revised set of "Magic Six" stretches in his columns and in his book *Running to Win* (Rodale Press, 1991). The following is a slightly modified version of Dr. Sheehan's Magic Six, Plus Two.

1. The *wall pushup* is a calf stretch that stretches one leg at a time. Stand with your rear foot approximately 2–3 feet from the wall. Your rear leg should be straight, your front leg bent, and your hands against the wall. Point your feet straight ahead and keep your heels on the ground. Hold for 30 seconds, then switch legs.
2. Next is the *hamstring stretch*: Straighten one leg, placing it with knee locked on a foot stool. Bend forward at your waist and bring your head toward your leg. Hold this position for 30 seconds and then switch sides.
3. A good stretch for a tight lower back is the *knee clasp*. Lie face up on a firm surface (a carpeted floor or on grass is best). Bring both knees to your chest and hold for 30 seconds.
4. Another excellent stretch is the *prone press-up*. Lie face down on the floor with your abdomen pressed flat against the floor. Place your hands flat on the floor, beneath your shoulders. Relax your abs and push up by straightening your arms (this will arch your back) and hold for 30 seconds.
5. To do the *backward stretch*, you simply place the palms of your hands against the small of your back while standing straight. Tighten your buttocks, and bend backward. Hold for 30 seconds.
6. The *shin splinter* is an exercise to strengthen the shin muscles. Sit on a table with your legs dangling over the side. Attach a 3- to 5-pound weight

to your forefoot. Flex your foot at the ankle (bending it up). Hold for 6 seconds then lower your foot; repeat 20 to 30 times.

7. To strengthen the quadriceps, do *straight-leg lifts*. Lying on the floor, bend one knee at approximately a right angle. Move the other leg rapidly up and down from 30–60 degrees. Lower and repeat ten times. Switch legs, repeat five times, and work up to ten sets of ten repetitions.

8. Finally, the *bent-leg sit-up* strengthens the abdominals. Dr. Sheehan recommends the sit-up be a gradual bending forward, one vertebrae at a time. Lie on the floor with your knees bent. Sit up at a 30-degree angle from the floor. Lie back, and then repeat twenty times. Do not hook your feet under anything to hold them down. If your spine is stiff, you may not be able to do this exercise.

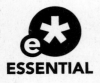

ESSENTIAL

Since hardly any runner wants to perform eight stretches (even if disguised as six plus two!), the four exercises you should do for optimal health and injury prevention are the wall pushup, hamstring stretch, knee clasp, and bent-leg sit-up.

Avoid Overstretching

Even as many runners neglect stretching, some in fact overstretch, perhaps in response to injury. This is usually not a good thing.

An example of when overstretching can be harmful involves stretching a strained muscle. A muscle strain is nothing more than a tear of the muscle fibers. If you are suffering from a strained muscle, stretching must be done *very* gently or else you risk tearing the muscle fibers even more. Stretching should *not* increase pain in the sore muscle. Give your injured muscle the best opportunity to heal by avoiding rigorous stretching.

The Biomechanics of Foot and Leg Problems

To understand lower-leg problems that runners encounter, you should be aware of how biomechanical abnormalities in the lower body are related to specific foot and leg problems. The following is a review of the gait cycle, which leads to a more complex discussion of foot and lower-leg biomechanics.

Many specific foot problems are caused by biomechanical faults within the foot or lower leg. In order to understand the cause of these problems, it helps to have a working knowledge of the normal anatomy, function, and biomechanics of the lower leg. By visualizing the events of the normal gait cycle during walking or running and breaking these down into phases and subphases, each action of the foot and leg can be evaluated at a specific sequential time period.

Anatomy of the Gait

Before understanding the specifics of gait, let's take a brief look at the bones involved. The key bone structures involved are the *talus* and *calcaneus* (located at the ankle and comprising the subtalar joint) and the *navicular* and *cuboid* (located in the midfoot just forward of the ankle). The talus and navicular along with the calcaneus and cuboid make up what is known as the *midtarsal* joint. The leg bones of significance consist of the *femur* (thigh bone) and the *tibia* (the larger of the two lower-leg bones). The *fibula* is the smaller lower-leg bone. The kneecap is called the *patella*.

Phases of Gait

The gait cycle of each leg is divided into the *stance phase* and the *swing phase*. The stance phase is the period during which the foot is in contact with the ground; the swing phase is the period in which the foot is off the ground and swinging forward.

FACT

It is important to note that in running a third subphase is present called the *float phase*. During the float phase, neither foot is on the ground. This is what differentiates walking from running. Walking has no float phase; one foot is always in contact with the ground when you're walking.

In walking, the stance phase comprises approximately 60 percent of the gait cycle and the swing phase about 40 percent. The proportion of swing to stance phase changes as the speed of walking or running increases. As the speed is increased, the percentage of time spent in the stance phase decreases. Increased time is then spent in the swing phase, with a corresponding increase in the importance of swing phase muscles.

Stance and Swing Phases of Gait

The stance phase comprises 40 percent of the gait cycle in running, compared with 60 percent of the gait cycle in walking. The time period during which forces are applied also differs dramatically between running and walking. A walker moving at a comfortable speed of 120 steps per minute has a total gait cycle time of 1 second. A runner moving at 12 miles per hour has a cycle time of 0.6 second, even though the stance phase decreases from .62 second to 0.2 seconds.

The stance phase can be further subdivided into three subphases. The first is called *heel contact*, which begins when the heel makes contact with the ground and is completed when the remainder of the foot touches the ground. During this portion of the stance phase, the foot is pronating at the *subtalar joint*. The leg is internally rotating while the foot is absorbing shock and functioning as a mobile adaptor to the ground surface.

The next portion of the stance phase is called *midstance*, which begins when the entire foot contacts the ground. The body weight passes over the foot as the tibia and the rest of the body move forward. The opposite leg is off the ground and the foot bears the body weight alone. During this subphase, the leg is externally rotating and the foot is supinating at the subtalar joint. The foot changes from being a mobile adaptor to becoming a rigid lever in order to propel the body forward during the final component of the stance phase, known as *propulsion*.

Propulsion begins after the heel is off the ground (heel off) and ends when the toe is off the ground (toe off). This subphase constitutes the final 35 percent of stance phase. The body is propelled forward during this subphase while weight is shifted to the opposite foot as it makes ground contact. The subtalar joint must be in a supinated position in order for this subphase to be normal and efficient. If abnormal pronation is occurring, the midstance subphase and this propulsion subphase are probably prolonged, with the result that weight transfer through the fore-foot is not normal.

The swing phase begins immediately after toe-off. The first component of the swing phase is the *forward swing,* which occurs as the foot is being carried forward. The knee is flexed, and the ankle is dorsiflexed (lifting up) at this time. The next segment is called *foot descent,* in which the foot is positioned for weight bearing and the muscles stabilize the body to absorb the shock of heel contact. At heel contact the swing phase ends, and a new gait cycle begins.

In normal walking, the foot initially contacts the ground at the heel. The major determinant of where maximum heel wear occurs is the initial point of contact as determined by the transverse plane position of the foot at the time of contact. Medial heel wear likely indicates a gait in which the toes point in and usually occurs when there is rotational abnormality in the limb.

In the gait of much faster speeds, such as sprinting, there may be no initial heel contact. An individual might make contact at midfoot and then rock backward onto the heel or not touch the heel down at all.

FACT

During running, if a runner swings his arms across his body, there is a compensatory increase in pelvic rotation. It is more efficient for the pelvis and better for the pelvic musculature if the runner moves his arms parallel to the motion in which he is running.

Selecting a Sports Physician

When selecting a physician to treat a running injury, it is important to choose a doctor with experience in treating athletes. You cannot rely on finding such a doctor simply by looking in a telephone book. Your best source of information is other runners. Ask around; chances are high that several members of an area running club have needed treatment from a specialist sports doctor. A specialty running store is another source since the employees there typically are runners. Even if they're not, they should be able to put you in touch with individuals or groups that can help you. Why go to all this trouble? Because it is vital that you choose a medical specialist with both experience and a good reputation among runners.

QUESTION

Should the sports physician be a runner, too?
Whether the doctor is also a runner doesn't matter. Although a doctor-athlete can add to your understanding of the physical conditions that lead to injury, this is not a prerequisite for appropriate diagnosis and treatment. The recommendations of knowledgeable people are the most valuable resource for finding a capable sports medicine physician.

Board Certification

A primary care physician can pursue specialized *primary care* sports medicine training and can obtain a "Certificate of Added Qualifications (CAQ) in sports medicine." For this certificate, the doctor attends a one- to two-year sports medicine fellowship then sits for a rigorous examination. A physician who completes an orthopedic surgery residency may also do a *surgical* sports medicine fellowship, which lasts one to two additional years and become "board certified" in sports medicine.

Two organizations grant "board certification" and "certificate of added qualifications" certifications: the American Board of Medical Specialties (ABMS), and the American Osteopathic Association (AOA) Bureau of Osteopathic Specialists. Sports medicine certifications can also be obtained by other physician professional organizations. The American Board of Family Medicine administers an examination that is then used for sports certification by the American Board of Emergency Medicine, American Board of Pediatrics, and the American Board of Internal Medicine.

To locate a primary care sports medicine doctor in your area, you can contact the American Medical Society for Sports Medicine (AMSSM) or the American Osteopathic Academy of Sports Medicine (AOASM).

CHAPTER 13

Injuries of the Foot and Ankle

It is beyond the scope or authority of this book to discuss in detail the nature and treatment of most running injuries. For best results, you should work with a trusted sports physician to determine the appropriate course of treatment. However, in order to give a practical overview of as many common injuries as possible, this chapter focuses alphabetically on injuries of the foot and ankle.

General Injury Guidelines

Should you run with an injury? Perhaps, so long as you can run at a level of intensity below the threshold of pain without altering your normal running stride. When an injury occurs, at the very least, reduce your mileage and intensity until you can resume running without pain. Do not take medication or ice an injury before testing whether or not you can run without pain, since doing so would only mask the injury and possibly make it worse.

ALERT

> If something hurts, do not run; instead, choose a cross-training activity to maintain cardiovascular fitness. The following sports are generally safe for injured runners but check with your doctor for clearance: walking, elliptical training, cycling, swimming, deep-water running, rowing, yoga, and Pilates. If you must stop running altogether for more than a week, ease back into your running slowly.

Recognize the difference between fatigue and pain due to an injury. Unfortunately, feel-good endorphins (the chemicals the body produces from aerobic exercise) mask pain. Listen to your body, and respect what it is telling you.

Some minor discomforts go away once muscles warm up. Be very cautious in this case, for you don't want to cause more serious damage to an injury site. Above all, if pain becomes more intense while running, do not continue. Stop and walk and then begin treating the injury when you get home.

Achilles Tendonitis

Achilles tendonitis is the bane of many runners. The Achilles tendon connects the heel with the most powerful muscle group in the body, located in the back of your lower leg. The tendon is the hard cord that you feel behind your ankle. The Achilles tendon is the common tendon for two muscles—the double-headed *gastrocnemius* and the *soleus*. Together these calf muscles are responsible for raising you up onto your toes (plantar flexion) and pushing off while you run and walk.

The gastrocnemius is a muscle that crosses two joints: the knee and the ankle. The functioning of these joints and the influence of other muscles on these joints has a significant effect on the tension that occurs within the Achilles tendon. For example, tight hamstrings impact the functioning of the ankle joint and the subtalar joint, and increase tension in the Achilles tendon.

FACT

The Achilles tendon does not have a rich blood supply. The blood supply to the proximal portion of the tendon comes from the branches of the calf muscles themselves. Because of this, the tendon is slower to heal, which drags out an Achilles tendon injury or tendonitis.

What Causes Achilles Tendonitis

Chronic Achilles tendonitis arises from ignoring pain in your Achilles tendon and continuing to run while injured. Tendonitis is the inflammation of the tendon. It is this tendonitis that causes the pain. If your Achilles tendon is getting sore, you should attend to it immediately.

Sudden increases in training can cause Achilles tendonitis, particularly excessive hill running or a sudden addition of hills and speed work.

ALERT

A major contributor to Achilles tendonitis is excessive tightness of the posterior leg muscles—the calf muscles and the hamstrings. If your Achilles tendon is sore, perform only gentle calf stretching. Excessive stretching is not good for your Achilles tendon. In most cases, stretches put too much tension on an already tender Achilles tendon.

Two shoe construction flaws can also aggravate Achilles tendonitis. The first is a sole that is too stiff, especially at the ball of the foot. This means the "lever arm" of the foot is longer and the Achilles tendon is under increased tension, forcing the calf muscles to work harder to lift your heel off the ground.

The second shoe factor that can lead to a chronic Achilles tendon problem is excessive heel cushioning. Air-filled heels, which supposedly are now more resistant to deformation and leaks, are not good for a sore Achilles tendon. The reason for this is quite simple. If you are wearing a shoe designed to give superior heel shock absorption, what frequently happens is that after heel contact, your heel continues to sink lower while your shoe is absorbing the shock. This further stretches the Achilles tendon at a moment when the leg and the rest of the body are moving forward over the foot. So, change your shoes to one without this feature. Make sure to avoid training in racing flats if you have Achilles tendonitis.

Treating Achilles Tendonitis

If you are suffering from Achilles tendonitis, the first thing to do is to cut back on your training. If you are working out twice a day, change to once a day and take one or two days off per week. If you are working out every day, cut back to every other day and decrease your mileage. Training modification is *essential* to treatment of this potentially long-lasting problem. You should also cut back on hill work and speed work.

Applying ice after running is also very important. Icing is an anti-inflammatory treatment, and remember, tendonitis is an inflammation issue. Be sure to avoid excessive stretching. Accompany the first phase of healing with relative rest, which doesn't necessarily mean stopping running but just cutting back in training. If this does not help quickly, consider adding a quarter-inch heel lift into your shoe. Do not worry that you will become dependent on this; instead, concentrate on getting rid of the pain. Don't walk barefoot around your house and avoid excessively flat shoes.

Clinical treatment of Achilles tendonitis initially consists of the physical therapy manual techniques and possibly modalities such as electrical stimulation and ultrasound. Your sports physician or physical therapist should also carefully check your shoes. Supportive shoe inserts such as Superfeet® can help control excessive pronation. These methods can be incorporated in a program of Achilles tendonitis rehabilitation therapy that also includes gentle stretching and graded strengthening exercise. Orthotics with a small heel lift are often helpful. A resting night splint can be used for tough cases.

When the Achilles Tendon Ruptures

Although relatively uncommon, a ruptured or torn Achilles tendon is a very serious and potentially permanently debilitating injury that may require a surgical repair and casting or splinting to properly heal. If you suspect this has happened to you, read carefully and consult a trusted sports physician as soon as possible.

What actually causes the Achilles tendon to rupture is not entirely known, though it is associated with overworking unused or overused muscles. It is an injury common to the weekend warrior who doesn't exercise consistently but may overexercise on the weekend. It can happen to seasoned athletes too. The mechanism of injury is a force that increases the tension in the Achilles tendon beyond its tensile strength. A forceful stretch of the tendon or a contraction of the muscles can create this force. Most often it is a combination of the two forces.

Occasionally, ruptures occur at the tendon-bone interface or within a 3- to 5-centimeter area above the tendon's insertion point on the heel. Since vascularity decreases with age, this frequently occurs in older athletes. A weakening of the Achilles tendon has been observed following intratendinous steroid injection. Therefore, injections of steroids are not recommended at this location. Diseases associated with an increased incidence of tendon rupture include gout, systemic lupus erythematosus, rheumatoid arthritis, and tuberculosis.

Diagnosing a Ruptured Achilles

The cardinal signs of a ruptured Achilles tendon are severe heel pain and the inability to walk. Physical examination of the site of a recent rupture may reveal a noticeable gap. Swelling is observed. The most frequently prescribed clinical test is called the Thompson test: As you lie on your stomach, your calf is squeezed. If your foot plantar-flexes then you do *not* have a completely torn Achilles tendon. However, if the foot does not plantar-flex when the calf is squeezed, chances are the Achilles tendon is completely torn. An MRI will accurately reveal the extent of the tear. Diagnostic ultrasound is also used to assist in the diagnosis of a torn Achilles tendon.

Treating a Ruptured Achilles Tendon

Complete tears of the Achilles tendon are usually treated with surgical repair followed by up to twelve weeks in a series of casts. Partial tears are sometimes treated with casting alone for up to twelve weeks or are sometimes treated as complete tears, with surgery and casting. A heel lift is usually used for six months to one year following removal of the cast. Following cast removal, rehabilitation with a physical therapist is necessary to regain your flexibility and muscle strength and also to restore your normal walking and eventually your running gait.

Ankle Sprains

Ankle sprains are more common in athletes participating in sports with side-to-side movement than in those with straight-ahead motion. Court sports such as basketball, tennis, and racquetball all spawn their fair share of ankle sprains. Running on level ground does not often result in an ankle sprain, but cross-country running, trail running, stepping in a pothole, or missing the curb can all potentially lead to an ankle sprain. The most frequent ankle sprain is an inversion ankle sprain, in which your arch turns inwards. This can injure the outer (lateral) structures of the ankle.

The most common ankle injury resulting from an inversion is a partial tear of the *anterior talofibular ligament* (ATFL). This ligament can be partially torn or may also tear completely. The next most frequently injured ligament is the *calcaneofibular ligament*. The least injured is the *posterior talofibular ligament*. On occasion, the fibula itself may be fractured or the talar dome injured. The other structures on the lateral side of the ankle should always be carefully examined to make sure they are not injured.

The grading of ankle sprains is done using a three-point scale. Grade 1 is a mild stretch of ligament(s), Grade 3 is a complete tear of ligament(s), and Grade 2 is everything in between.

Treatment for Ankle Sprains

It is impossible to guess how badly injured you are. If you have doubts or if your ankle swells very rapidly, you should head for an emergency room. Immediate treatment should consist of RICE: Rest, Ice, Compression (gentle), and Elevation of the limb. The ice (or a cold pack) should be applied for about 15 minutes at a time and then removed for at least the same amount of time. A bag of frozen corn or peas also works well. If your ankle does not respond quickly to this treatment, it is probably best to visit your sports physician for an evaluation and treatment.

For Grade 2 sprains, an air cast is sometimes recommended to hold the ankle still to prevent further tearing or strain as it heals. A removable walking cast is used for the more serious sprains to provide stability and security while allowing you to bear weight without pain.

Starting to Exercise the Injury

The first exercise to try once your ankle starts to feel better is dorsiflexion–plantar flexion, or just plain moving the foot up and down (called an ankle pump). Progress to performing such things as moving your foot in small circles and painting the alphabet with your toes. Later still, you can use an exercise band and perform other exercises to strengthen the muscles that control your ankle. Don't force your ankle to move in pain too soon, and avoid weight bearing or walking in pain early in the course of an ankle sprain. You might need to walk with a cane or crutch. There is no reason to start testing your ankle until it has had time to heal. "Slow and easy" gains more than rushing into painful exercises. One way to see if you are ready to resume your full exercise regimen is to try walking down stairs, hopping, or jumping rope. Before attempting to run again, you must be able to walk for at least 20 minutes without limping, pain, or limitation. For Grade 2 and Grade 3 ankle sprains, physical therapy treatment may be necessary to restore your full range of motion, strength, proprioception, and to help you to safely return to running.

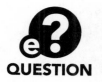

QUESTION

What is the best way to apply ice to an injury?
Ice can be applied to an injured area in the form of a bag of ice (crushed is best), a cold pack, or a bag of tiny frozen vegetables such as corn or peas. Ice the painful area for 15–20 minutes at a time. For best results, put the ice right against your skin. If you cannot tolerate the ice directly on your skin, put the ice in a pillow case. Remove the ice once the injured area is numb. Leave the ice off for at least 40 minutes. You can safely ice an injury three to five times a day. Be careful, because you can get frostbite from leaving the ice on one area for too long.

Anterior Ankle Pain

The tendons in front of your ankle can sometimes become irritated when your shoes are laced too tightly. This can also compress the nerves in this area, resulting in occasional numbness, but most often the problem is pain. Of course, injuries to ligaments or bones can also cause pain in this area. Try skipping the top lace completely rather than lacing it looser. You can then lace your shoe securely without irritation. Odds are this should help a lot. If this simple solution doesn't work, have your foot examined by a sports medicine practitioner.

Athlete's Foot

You don't have to be an athlete to have athlete's foot (tinea pedis). The condition got its name because it is spread in warm, moist places such as locker rooms. Athlete's foot is actually caused by a fungus or a type of mold, less often by a yeast. Fungus flourishes in dark, warm, moist environments. Shoes, being an occlusive covering of the foot, can be like a fungal heaven.

Clinical Appearance of Athlete's Foot

Athlete's foot can appear as cracked and peeling skin between the toes or on the bottom of the foot. It is often itchy but not always. Sometimes the flaking, scaling, or dry skin that you think is just a bit of excessive dryness is in reality evidence of athlete's foot. Small blisters may occur in conjunction with some fungal infections.

Between the toes the skin can become macerated or excessively soft and mushy. The fungus can go deeper into the skin through cracks or breaks, so that bacteria enters and causes a more troubling secondary bacterial infection.

Preventing Athlete's Foot

As with many things, the best cure is prevention. Since moisture is a risk factor, keeping your feet dry is important. Make sure you dry your feet carefully after showers. In the locker room, consider wearing shower sandals to limit exposure to any areas contaminated with fungus. Be careful to dry between your toes, and make sure your feet are dry before putting on your socks. You might sprinkle an antifungal foot powder in your shoes or on your feet.

Another important thing to remember is that cotton socks hold moisture against the foot rather than allowing it to readily evaporate. It is best to wear socks made of non-cotton material that wicks moisture away from the foot.

Treating Athlete's Foot

Mild fungal infections can be treated with over-the-counter medicine readily found in your pharmacy. Stubborn fungal infections require prescription-strength medicine. Make certain you follow directions for prevention to avoid a recurrence and to speed up elimination of the fungal infection. Keeping your feet dry is key to eliminating and preventing re-infection.

Plantar Fasciitis and Heel Spurs

The most common heel problems are actually caused by a painful irritation or tearing of the plantar fascia. Damage to the plantar fascia can result in plantar fasciitis, which, over time, may lead to a heel spur.

If your foot flattens or becomes unstable during critical times in the walking or running cycle, the attachment of the plantar fascia to your heel bone may begin to stretch and pull away. This will result in inflammation, pain, and possibly swelling. The pain is especially noticeable when you push off with your toes while walking, since this movement stretches the already inflamed tissue. The bottom of the heel can also be exquisitely tender to pressure.

Without treatment, the pain will usually spread along the arch of your foot and around your heel. The pain is usually centered just in front of the heel toward the arch. When the tearing occurs at the bone itself, the bone may attempt to heal itself by producing new bone. This results in the development of a heel spur. Heel spurs are visible on X-rays, which is how their existence is confirmed.

The pain of this condition can cause you to walk on your toes or alter your running stride and gait, which can cause further damage. Gait changes in running and walking can also lead to pain in a remote location such as your knee, hip, back, or sometimes in your opposite leg.

Causes of Heel Spurs and Plantar Fasciitis

The most frequent cause of these injuries is excessive pronation. Normally, while walking or during long-distance running, your foot will strike the ground on the heel, then roll forward toward your toes and inward to the arch. Your arch should only dip slightly during this motion. If it lowers too much, you will have excessive pronation.

The mechanical structure of your feet and the manner in which the different segments of your feet are linked together and joined with your legs has a major effect on their function and on the development of mechanically caused problems. Having badly functioning feet with poor bone alignment will adversely affect the muscles, ligaments, and tendons, and can create a variety of aches and pains. Excess pronation can cause the arch of your foot to stretch excessively with each step. It can also cause too much motion in segments of the foot that should be stable as you are walking or running. This hypermobility may cause other bones to shift that may lead to other mechanically induced problems.

Other factors that can contribute to plantar fasciitis and heel spurs include a sudden increase in daily activities, an increase in weight (not usually a problem with runners), or a change of shoes. Dramatic increase in training intensity or duration (training errors) also can cause plantar fasciitis.

Treatment of Plantar Fasciitis

As with most running-related injuries, evaluate any changes in your training. A decrease in workout intensity and duration is important. Self-treatment for this condition entails applying ice to the painful area and to gently stretch your calf. Make sure that your shoes offer motion control so they're not contributing to plantar fasciitis and heel spurs.

Check your running shoes to make sure they are not excessively worn or too stiff. They should bend only at the ball of the foot, where your toes attach to the foot. This is vital! Avoid any shoe that bends in the center of the arch or behind the ball of the foot. It offers insufficient support and will stress your plantar fascia. The human foot was not designed to bend here, and neither should a shoe be designed to do this.

If self-treatment fails, pay a visit to a sports physician and then to a physical therapist. The physical therapist may use manual (hands on) techniques to address alignment problems or hypomobility issues in your foot, ankle, or leg. He may also use modalities such as laser light, ultrasound, and electrical stimulation. The physical therapist may also make recommendations on devices such as a night splint or Strassburg Sock®.

ESSENTIAL

Perform the shoe pushup test to check where your shoe ends. Hold the heel of the shoe in one hand and then press up underneath the forefoot. The shoe should bend at the ball of the shoe, where the metatarsals would be. Next press under the part of the shoe where the metatarsal heads would be. The shoe should not bend under moderate pressure in this area.

Following control of the pain and inflammation associated with plantar fasciitis, you may need an orthotic to stabilize your foot and prevent a recurrence. The orthotic prevents excess pronation and prevents lengthening of the plantar fascia and continued tearing of the fascia. Usually a slight heel lift and a firm shank in the shoe will also help to reduce the severity of this problem.

More than 98 percent of the time, heel spurs and plantar fasciitis can be controlled by this type of treatment, and surgery can be avoided.

Morton's Neuroma Pain

Morton's neuroma pain, sometimes referred to simply as neuroma pain, is classically described as a burning pain in the forefoot. It can also be felt as an aching or shooting pain in this area. You might feel like you want to take off your shoes and rub your foot. It may occur in the middle of a run or at the end of a long run. If your shoes are quite tight it may occur very early in the run. The pain can usually be re-created by compressing the toes together by squeezing the forefoot.

Causes of Neuroma Pain

The source of this neuroma pain is an enlargement of the sheath of an intermetatarsal nerve in the foot. This usually occurs in the space between the third and fourth toes and metatarsals, which is where this particular nerve is thickest.

Pronation of the foot can cause the metatarsal heads to rotate slightly and pinch the nerve that runs between the metatarsal heads. This chronic pinching can make the nerve sheath enlarge. As it enlarges, it becomes more squeezed and increasingly troublesome.

Treating Neuromas

Treatment of this condition is mostly practical, having a lot to do with your shoes. It includes wearing shoes with a wide toebox, not lacing the forefoot part of your shoe too tightly, and making sure your feet are in supportive shoes but not being squeezed. If this doesn't relieve the pain, work with a doctor to decide on these treatments: orthotics, an injection of steroids, or surgical removal of the neuroma, preferably in that order.

CHAPTER 14

Injuries of the Leg and Other Areas

As previously stated, it is beyond the scope and authority of this book to provide detailed information about treatments. Every injury is unique, and, again, for best results, you should work with a trusted sports physician to determine the appropriate course of treatment. This chapter provides an overview of injuries of the leg and other areas affected by running, listed in alphabetical order.

Anterior Shin Splints

The medical term *anterior shin splints* was replaced several years ago. Now the symptoms that occur in the anterior lateral tibial region (the front of your shin, anterior meaning front side) are assumed to be either stress fractures or a form of compartment syndrome. In understanding the anterior shin splint, it is therefore important to differentiate a shin splint from a stress fracture.

Most injuries that fit the term anterior shin splint are soft-tissue injuries at the muscular origin and bony or periosteal interface of the bone and muscle origin. These usually result in a more vertical area of symptoms, that is, they tend to run up and down the front of your shin.

Most injuries that clinically seem to be stress fractures have what is called a region of pinpoint tenderness and extend in a horizontal direction (side to side at the pain site). This line in many stress fractures of the tibia extends horizontally but might take a tangential course through the tibia. For injuries that are horizontal, no tenderness is found 1 or 2 centimeters above or below this discrete line of tenderness.

The non-stress fracture type injury to this area is thought to be due to micro-tears of the muscle either at the site of attachment to the bone or in the muscle fibers themselves. This may occur because of repetitive traction or pulling of the anterior (front) tibial muscles at the attachment site. Repetitive loading with excessive stress, such as caused by running on concrete, may also play a role in injury to this area. This can result in micro-trauma to the bone structure itself.

Anterior Compartment Syndrome

The muscles in your body are all wrapped in tissue called fascia. This packaging of the muscles forms compartments that encloses the muscle and separates it from adjacent muscles. Anterior compartment syndrome is caused by the muscles swelling within a closed compartment, with a resultant increase in pressure. This running-related compartment syndrome is usually chronic, caused by repetitive stress, and is in some respects different from the acute compartment syndrome seen after serious muscle injuries. It is vital to seek medical evaluation and treatment if this condition is suspected. The blood supply can be compromised inside this compartment, resulting in muscle injury and pain. The symptoms include leg pain, unusual nerve sensations (paresthesia), and eventually, muscle weakness. Definitive evaluation measures the pressure in the compartment. In severe cases, surgical decompression of the compartment may be required to relieve pain.

Runners at Risk for Anterior Shin Splints

The usual runners at risk for anterior shin splints are beginning runners whose legs are not yet acclimated to the stresses of running. These runners also may not have been doing an adequate amount of stretching. Poor choice of shoes and running surface (such as concrete) can also play a role. Overtraining, of course, can be a factor, as it is with most running injuries.

The usual mechanical factor seen is an imbalance between the posterior (rear) and anterior (front) muscle groups. The posterior muscles of the calf may be both too tight and too strong. The effect of too tight posterior musculature has ramifications for the gait cycle at two points.

The first period in which too tight posterior muscles impact the anterior muscles is just before and after heel contact by the distance runner. At this time the anterior muscles are acting as decelerators. If the posterior muscles are too tight, they force the anterior muscles to work longer and harder in this deceleration.

The second point in the gait cycle at which the anterior muscles may work too hard is when the foot leaves the ground, just after toe-off. The anterior muscles should be lifting up, or dorsiflexing, the foot at this time so that the toes clear the ground as the leg is brought forward. If the posterior muscles are too tight, the anterior muscles again work harder than they should. Logically, downhill running also has an adverse effect on the anterior muscles. The anterior muscles are working to slow down the foot to keep it from slapping on the ground.

Repetitive impact on hard surfaces is another frequently associated factor. Excessive pronation may be a minor factor, though it is a much greater factor in medial shin splints (now called *medial tibial stress syndrome*, or MTSS). Overstriding during speed work in underconditioned runners can also contribute to this problem.

Self-Care

Decrease training immediately if you think you are experiencing these symptoms or conditions. Do not run if pain occurs during or following your run. Nonweight-bearing exercise may be necessary. Your goal is to find the distance you can run (if any) that does not produce symptoms, rather than to find your real limit. Swimming, biking, and deep-water running can all be used to maintain fitness.

It's recommended that you do gentle stretching of the calf muscles and the hamstrings. It is also important to be strengthening the muscles in the front of your shin.

Replace shoes with too many miles on them. Shock absorption should be a factor in selecting shoes if you suffer from anterior shin splints. Downhill running can aggravate this problem and should be avoided. A stride that's too long can also delay healing. Most of all, *do not run on concrete*. After exercise, apply ice to lessen symptoms.

Office Medical Care of Anterior Shin Splints

A thorough evaluation of your training and racing schedule and shoes is followed by a biomechanical evaluation. A bone scan can be used, if necessary, to evaluate the possibility of stress fracture. A wick catheter test can be used, if necessary, to measure post-exercise compartment pressure, if a compartment syndrome is suspected.

Anti-inflammatory medication can be prescribed. A physical therapy consultation and treatments can also be helpful to identify and treat the source of your specific problem.

Sometimes a heel lift is used to reduce the pulling effect of tight posterior muscles. Even though this increases the distance the foot must be dorsiflexed, the duration of action and the effective strength of the posterior muscles is decreased. Orthotics may also be considered when biomechanical abnormalities exist and problems persist.

Dry Heaves or Vomiting

Dry heaves have been associated with training that goes into the anaerobic (without oxygen) realm. If you feel dry heaves coming on at the end of your interval or race, slow down but keep moving. Don't stop. The movement will help keep your heart pumping, the blood flowing, and flush out some of the lactic acid buildup. Slowing down at the end of your workout also helps your body adapt to a more static state. A proper cool-down is always in order—good for the muscles, the body, and the soul. After that, you can hydrate and jump into the shower.

Iliotibial Band Syndrome

Symptoms of iliotibial band syndrome (ITBS), also called iliotibial band friction syndrome (ITBFS), are pain or aching on the outer side of the knee. This usually happens in the middle or at the end of a run. Factors contributing to this syndrome are weak hip abductor muscles, bow legs, pronation of the foot, leg length differences, and running on a banked (slanted) surface. Circular track running may also contribute to this problem since it stresses the body in a manner similar to that of crowned surfaces and leg length differences. Changes in training (often sudden increases in mileage) also frequently contribute to this problem.

Anatomy of the IT Band

The iliotibial band is a thickening of the soft tissue that envelops the lateral (outer) thigh. Its origin is at the top of the pelvis (iliac crest) and it attaches past the knee joint to the outer tibia. It receives fibers from two hip abductor muscles: the tensor fasciae latae (a muscle in the front of the hip) and the gluteus maximus (muscle in the buttocks). A bursa beneath the IT band is often the site of lateral knee pain in runners.

Treatment for IT Band Friction Syndrome

To self-treat this problem, you should:

- Temporarily decrease training
- Apply ice to the painful area
- Avoid crowned surfaces (roads) or too much running around a track
- Shorten your stride
- Wear more motion-control shoes to limit pronation (if necessary)

- Strengthen your hip abductor muscles (gluteus medius and tensor fasciae latae muscles)
- Carefully examine your training regimen (and running diary)

Some believe that proper stretching of the IT band is beneficial. The tendinous band itself is made of *collagen*, an inelastic, fibrous tissue that does not stretch. The hip abductors that attach to the IT band can be stretched, although tight abductors are not a cause of ITBFS—but *weak* hip abductors are a cause. So strengthening the abductors is more important than stretching them. If you do want to stretch them, here is one way: While standing, place your injured leg behind the good one. If the left side is the sore side, cross your left leg behind your right one. Then lean away from the injured side toward your right side. Lean on a table or chair for balance as you do this. Hold for 10–15 seconds, and repeat on each side three to five times. Be careful not to overstretch.

Hip abductor strengthening is best performed by lying on your side with your top leg straight and your bottom leg bent at the knee. Raise and lower your top leg with your foot aiming straight ahead. Perform two sets of 20 to 30 reps on each leg.

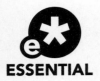

ESSENTIAL

If your self-treatment is not completely successful, then a trip to a sports medicine specialist may result in either a steroid injection beneath the IT band or a referral to physical therapy. Treatment is usually successful; this is not a career-ending injury, (although it may feel like one).

Medial Shin Splints—Now Called Medial Tibial Stress Syndrome (MTSS)

The outmoded term *medial shin splints* has been replaced by *medial tibial stress syndrome* (MTSS). Either term suffices to describe pain at the medial aspect of the leg, adjacent to the medial tibia. Tenderness is usually found between 3 and 12 centimeters above the tip of the *medial malleolus* (the inner knob of your ankle) along the tibia.

Periostitis (inflammation of the connective tissue that covers bone) sometimes occurs at the painful site. The sore, inflamed structures also usually include the adjacent muscles and tendons.

Stress fractures can also occur in this same area. The definitive test for stress fracture is a bone scan, but false negatives and false positives sometimes occur because of the soft tissue and periosteal involvement in this injury. A physician's clinical examination is used to differentiate between medial tibial stress syndrome (MTSS) and a stress fracture. With MTSS, the tenderness extends along a considerable vertical distance of the tibia. When a stress fracture is present, tenderness usually extends horizontally across the inside and front of the tibia.

Risk Factors for MTSS

The first risk factor is overtraining. Evaluate your schedule to determine what training errors you may have made. Mechanically, overpronation is most likely to be the culprit. When the foot pronates too much, the medial structures of the leg are stretched and stressed, which increases the likelihood of injury. Running on a cambered surface, such as the side of a crowned road, can put the upper leg at risk to develop this problem because the corresponding foot is functioning in a pronated position.

Treating MTSS

Decrease training immediately. Do not run if pain occurs during or following your run. Nonweight-bearing exercise such as swimming, biking, and deep-water running may be necessary to maintain fitness. Although running on soft surfaces has been recommended for this problem, it is not likely to help a pure MTSS. The foot is more likely to pronate excessively on mushy grass or sand. Packed dirt is ideal, and avoiding concrete is also helpful.

In many cases, shoes rated high for control of pronation might help. Gentle calf stretching exercises are important, but control of pronation is more direct. Ice applications following running can offer some pain relief but are not curative. If symptoms persist, it is important to seek professional medical attention.

In the doctor's office, a thorough medical evaluation of your training schedule, racing schedule, and shoes is followed by a biomechanical evaluation. Anti-inflammatory medication can be prescribed. The use of physical therapy modalities and skilled interventions can also be helpful to treat this problem. Excessive pronation, which is a major contributing factor to this syndrome, can be corrected by the right running shoe, an over-the-counter shoe insert such as Superfeet®, or possibly custom orthotics.

Runner's Knee

The knee is a complex joint. It connects the tibia and femur (leg and thigh) and the patella (kneecap). One of the most common knee problems in running involves what is called the patello-femoral complex, the quadriceps muscles, kneecap, and patellar tendon. *Chondromalacia patella* (CMP) syndrome—what is called "runner's knee"—is a softening of the cartilage of the kneecap. Cartilage does not have the good blood supply that bone does, so when cartilage is damaged, it has trouble healing.

Causes of Runner's Knee

During running, certain mechanical conditions can predispose you to a mistracking kneecap. Portions of the cartilage may then be under either too much or too little pressure, and the appropriate intermittent compression needed for waste removal and nutrition supply to the knee may not be present. This can result in cartilage deterioration, which at the knee usually occurs on the medial aspect, or inner part of the kneecap.

The symptoms of runner's knee include pain near the kneecap, usually at the medial (inner) portion and below it. Pain is usually felt upon standing after sitting for a long period of time with the knees bent. Running downhill and sometimes even walking down stairs can be followed by pain. When the knee is bent, there is increased pressure between the surface of the kneecap and the femur. This stresses the injured area and leads to pain.

Too large a *Q* (quadriceps) *angle* increases a person's chances of having runner's knee. The Q angle is an estimate, on average, of the effective angle at which the quadriceps makes its pull. Your Q angle is determined by drawing a line from the *anterior superior iliac spine* (the bump on your pelvis above and in front of your hip joint) to the center of your kneecap, and a second line from the center of your kneecap to where the tendon below your kneecap attaches to the shin bone, and determining the angle between the two lines. A normal Q angle is less than 12 degrees, while definitely abnormal is greater than 15 degrees. If the line-of-pull of the Q angle is too high, the patella will be pulled off track laterally.

Often adding to the strong lateral pull of the bulk of the quadriceps is a weak *vastus medialis*. This is the portion of the quadriceps that helps medially to stabilize the patella (kneecap). It runs along the inside portion of the thigh bone to join at the kneecap with the other three muscles making up the quadriceps. Mechanical conditions that contribute to runner's knee include:

- Wide hips (female runners), causing a large Q angle
- Knock-knees
- Unstable kneecap (*subluxing patella*)
- High kneecap (*patella alta*)
- Weak thigh muscle, especially vastus medialis
- Excessive pronation of the feet

Treating Runner's Knee

At the early stage of runner's knee, you should decrease running to lessen stress to this area and allow healing to begin. It is important to avoid downhill running, which *really* stresses the patello-femoral complex. Avoid performing exercises with the knee bent, such as the knee extension machine at the gym. When the knee is bent, the forces under the kneecap are increased. Since the vastus medialis muscle is most active during the final 30 degrees of extension of the knee, quad strengthening exercises should be performed over these final 30 degrees.

You should stretch tight posterior muscles. In many cases, tight calf or hamstring muscles make the foot pronate while running or walking. This pronation is accompanied by an internal rotation of the leg, which increases the Q angle and contributes to the lateral dislocation of the kneecap. You should wear running shoes that offer extra support. If you need further control of pronation, consider orthotics. Usually, trying to stretch the quadriceps itself is counterproductive. This is often done with the knee bent and puts compression forces on the undersurface of the kneecap. If you would like to stretch the quadriceps, stand near a wall and move your entire leg backward the way a ballerina does.

A physical therapist can assess your collection of biomechanical and structural faults and then develop a treatment individualized to your needs. He can use such things as manual therapy techniques, taping, exercise, and modalities to treat runner's knee.

FACT

The late George Sheehan, MD, sports medicine physician and philosopher, first popularized the practice of examining the foot when runner's knee occurs. It is also important to rule out other knee problems when knee pain occurs from running, rather than attributing every such pain as runner's knee.

"Shin Splints"

In the past, the medical term *shin splint* was used to diagnose almost all problems occurring in the lower leg. These included both bone and soft tissue problems and those that overlapped. Now doctors use the terms *medial tibial stress syndrome, compartment syndrome,* and *stress fracture* to describe injuries of the lower leg. These are discussed earlier in this chapter.

Defining the Problem

Most athletes refer to pain occurring either in the anterior or the medial portion of the leg as a shin splint. Problems that occur in the lateral aspect of the leg are usually either stress fractures of the fibula or peroneal tendon injuries following an inversion injury of the ankle. Posterior lower-leg pains are frequently injuries to the posterior muscle group at the *myotendinous junction* of the calf muscles and Achilles tendon, or early Achilles tendonitis.

Side Stitches

Side stitches are pains that occur usually in your abdomen or just under your ribs (most often on the right side) when running. In the past it was thought that the pain was due to an unconditioned diaphragm, food allergies (often milk), gas, or having just eaten before running. Side stitches happen more often with beginning runners or when a runner is out of shape. Today it is believed that the side stitch occurs due to the lack of oxygen (*ischemia*) in a portion of the colon. There is a piece of the colon that, at times, may not receive an adequate blood supply. During rigorous exercise, when blood is shunted away from the gut and diverted to the limbs to supply the muscles, pain is experienced in this portion of the colon that is starved for oxygen.

Controlling Side Stitches

When caused by lack of conditioning, the best thing to do for side stitches is to run slower and longer. Breathe fuller and try belly breathing, in which you allow your stomach to relax and push out as you inhale and then contract slightly as you exhale fully. Breathe rhythmically and make sure that you are not holding your breath.

Another breathing tactic consists of exhaling against resistance through pursed lips. Combined with belly breathing, this may be the best approach. Applying direct pressure to the side stitch sometimes helps. Another way of gaining temporary relief is to stretch your arms up while inhaling, imagining your breath coming in and soothing the side stitch.

CHAPTER 15

Ready for Racing: The 5K

The 5K offers an array of challenges to all levels of runners. Experienced runners may wish to improve their time from a previous race, whereas beginning runners might simply hope to finish the event. Regardless of your motivation, running the 5K is a goal that you can accomplish after just a few short weeks of training. By the time you complete the first training schedule, you'll be able at least to finish a 5K without months of intense preparation, even if you have to walk for part or all of it.

5K Basics

Today the 5K (5 kilometers) is a distance that's familiar to runners the world over. It is accepted internationally as the introductory distance for novice runners as well as the proving ground for more competitive runners (and every level in between). Its distance—3.1 miles—doesn't seem that long and isn't too difficult to train for. But like most things that appear simple at first, the 5K is a race distance that challenges even elite runners to return for more.

Usually, 5K races, along with longer distance events, are well organized and are most often sponsored by a variety of organizations that include running clubs, civic groups, municipal recreation departments, charitable foundations, local businesses, and major corporations. The focus of many races is to raise awareness of worthwhile causes, with proceeds from these events oftentimes funding charitable, cultural, and educational institutions. As part of the entry fee, many events provide a uniquely designed race T-shirt to its participants; these T-shirts frequently become coveted souvenirs.

You will find that 5K races are lots of fun and much like little running fairs. Along with post-race refreshments, participants sometimes receive free samples of running-related products. Information about upcoming races is also readily available. Oftentimes many vendors are present that feature wares such as running shoes, athletic apparel, and other running-related accessories. It is not uncommon for people to have some fun indulging in a little shopping either before or after the race.

Of course, you'll also see a lot of other runners at 5K events. They come alone, in pairs, or in groups, all from diverse backgrounds. Buddies, girlfriends, boyfriends, couples, and families all attend, and they all love running as well as socializing with fellow runners.

FACT

The larger 5K races across the United States typically include runners expos. These are good venues to find sales on the basics: shoes, shorts, singlets, socks, sunglasses, nutritional products, and more! You can reward yourself for competing in the event by supplementing your running wardrobe before you go home.

Race Strategy and Goal Setting

Goal setting is indeed important. Not only does it keep your training in focus, but it makes competing in races both fun and challenging. In the weeks prior to the race, think about three goals you'd be interested in accomplishing: an easily obtainable goal, a realistic yet moderately challenging goal, and an ultimate goal. Be realistic. For example, if you don't possess the genetic gift to run a sub-16-minute 5K, don't set that as your ultimate goal.

Some 5K goals include completing the entire event running, improving your time by 30 seconds to a full minute, or coming in under a specific time. By making sure these goals are realistic, you will avoid being disappointed and instead be satisfied or even thrilled with your performance. Above all, it's important to keep the event in perspective. Sure, races are competitive. Sure, you want to do your best. But remember that one of the great things about running is that you're ultimately competing with yourself. So keep a healthy perspective, give yourself an achievable goal, and keep the fun in the 5K.

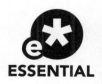

ESSENTIAL

While the tips presented in this section refer to participating in 5K and other short races, it's important to note that most of them can also be applied, at least in a general sense, to training for longer races, including 10Ks and half-marathons.

The Week Before Your 5K

There is no workout you can do in the last week prior to your 5K that will enhance your performance. Therefore, make the final week prior to the big race an easy one with light workouts (continue to follow either of the mileage buildup charts in Chapter 5). Make one of the two days prior to the event a complete leg rest day.

Don't try anything radically new or different in the weeks before your 5K. Don't try a new diet; don't try new shoes. Taper your mileage at an easy pace, get adequate rest, and prepare yourself mentally for the big day.

Don't break with your training schedule or try anything radically different the week before your race either. For example, one of the most frequent mistakes that comes back to haunt the unsuspecting runner, whether it be in a short event or in a marathon, is to run in new shoes purchased the day before the race. It takes at least a few training runs for new shoes to get broken in. Wearing new shoes even a few days before the race can cause a variety of problems, such as blisters and foot discomfort, which affects your performance in the race.

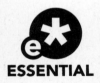

ESSENTIAL

Lay out everything you need (apparel, shoes, etc.) the evening before the race to save yourself time, stress, and aggravation in the morning. You don't want to be halfway to the race site and realize you've forgotten something, especially if you have to help others get ready to go with you. It's important to have everything you need arranged ahead of time.

What to Eat and Drink

Nutrition principles dictate that you should always stay well hydrated, whether you are exercising or not. In particular, drink ample fluids in the days prior to competition, regardless of how long the race may be, what the weather is like the day of the race, whether the course is particularly hilly, or other conditions of the race.

For workouts and races that last an hour or less, you need only drink water every 25–30 minutes to stay well hydrated. Although sports drinks do play an important role during runs lasting an hour and longer, they won't necessarily give you a performance edge for shorter workouts and events such as the 5K. Consuming sports drinks can be especially helpful when training in hot and humid conditions, however, as they refuel your body's electrolyte stores.

Eating Before Race Day

Carbohydrate loading and eating in general is a major consideration in running, whether to fuel your body for training runs or for a road race. However, you really don't need to load up too much on carbohydrates the day or two before a 5K, not in the same way you do for a marathon.

Don't stuff yourself, thinking you're just going to burn off the calories the next day. And don't eat new foods you haven't eaten during your training. Many a runner has regretted the time he decided to have exotic or unfamiliar food the day before a race. Eat something you know will agree with you. Otherwise, regardless of your pace, the consequence of poor nutritional choice can be discomforting and perhaps even embarrassing.

ESSENTIAL

If you're like many runners, you live for your next meal. Well, plan your eating extravagance for the night *after* the 5K. Leading up to the event, be mindful of any unnecessary fat, sugar, or other nutritional bombs that might put you in the bathroom instead of on the starting line come race day.

In summary, your evening meal the day before the race should consist of well-balanced and simple foods that you know will cause no digestive troubles. Avoid foods that are high in salt, fat, or are fried. You also want to limit your intake of foods with high roughage content, such as salads, vegetables, and cereals.

Drinking Before Race Day

As stressed throughout this book, stay well hydrated. If you enjoy beverages that contain caffeine such as coffee or tea, be aware that drinking these in late afternoon or evening may make it difficult for you to fall asleep easily, especially if you have pre-race jitters. Additionally, alcoholic beverages are diuretics that can contribute to dehydration.

At the other extreme, if you're taking in excessive fluids through water or sports drinks, you may experience hyponatremia, or water intoxication, a condition in which excess fluids create an imbalance between the body's water and sodium levels. This can lead to nausea, fatigue, vomiting, or worse.

Eating on Race Day

Equally important is your decision regarding what to eat on race day. If the race is set for early in the morning (as most 5Ks are), you may wish to bypass breakfast and just stick with water. If you choose to eat a light snack (this could be a banana, slice of toast, bagel, or energy bar), be sure to consume it at least 1 hour before the start of the race.

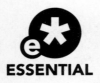

ESSENTIAL

Try to go to bed early the night prior to the race so you will be well rested for the event. You don't want to be rushed or, worse, oversleep and miss the race. Wake up early enough to eat, make a bathroom visit, and take care of anything you need to do so as not to feel rushed.

Events held during the late morning, midafternoon, or evening are more difficult to plan for nutritionally. While you certainly don't want to go hungry in the hours prior to a race or a fast-paced workout, you don't want to eat foods that cause stomach cramps or digestive problems.

Light, healthy snacks are your best approach for late morning and early afternoon races. If the race will be held in the evening, eat a healthy and satisfying breakfast along with a sensible but light lunch (avoid high-fat and fried foods). A piece of fruit or a handful of pretzels are good snack choices later in the afternoon. In short, the best way to determine which foods and fluids work best for you, whether during training runs or races, is by experimenting with these in practice.

Physical Preparation

Listen to your body. As mentioned previously, there are no workouts the week prior to any distance race that can enhance your preparedness. A general rule of thumb is that less is best. The physiological effects of training don't kick in for a week to ten days, so the workout you do today will not immediately enhance your level of performance.

Remember also not to try anything new the week prior to and during your 5K. There are so many heartbreaking stories of runners who tried something new in the week prior to a race, only to injure themselves and not be able to participate in the event at all. Don't let that happen to you.

The following are some 5K pre-race reminders:

- Preregister for the event to save time and money.
- Remember that the race will begin on time and regardless of almost any weather conditions (except perhaps lightning storms).
- Arrive at the race site early.
- Pin your race number on the front of your shirt or singlet.
- For computer-timed races, be sure that your computer chip is attached securely to your running shoe (for example, on an eyelet or on laces located midway down the tongue).

Psychological Issues and Concerns

Remember that it is normal to be tense or nervous prior to a road race of any distance. Even the most seasoned runners experience these feelings. To help yourself stay calm and focused, avoid spending too much time with participants who are excessively stressed out or negative. These individuals may adversely affect your state of mind—something you certainly don't need. If you find being in the company of others prior to an event comforting, gravitate toward those who appear focused and relaxed. Some runners find it calming to spend a few moments alone. Through racing you'll figure out what works best for you.

Prior to the start of the event, you'll notice a variety of pre-race activity. You'll see some runners stretching, some doing pre-race warm-up running, some taking in extra fluids. Don't second-guess yourself and think you should be doing any of these for a competitive advantage. If you try doing something different from your tried-and-true warm-up routine because you see others doing it, it may backfire on you during the race. Relax, do what you've rehearsed during your training, and feel good about it.

ALERT

Don't overpack when going to a race. Between the freebies you're given at the race and the goods you'll want to buy, you may have a lot to carry. If you're walking to the race, take a small bag that can be checked at the start. If you drive to the race, you can put your items in your car.

During the Race

As you are running the 5K, it's easy to get caught up in the excitement of it all. Just be sure that you keep the following essential guidelines in mind to ensure that you have the best experience possible.

The Start

When runners line up in anticipation at the start of a 5K (or any race), they are supposed to position themselves in the pack based on their antici-pated pace. For example, faster runners—especially those trying to place, if not win—line up in front to be sure they get off to as fast a start as possi-ble. Runners with no competitive aspirations, or those who are participating strictly for fun, should take their place toward the back.

Although runners generally are honest people, this protocol does not always hold when they are asked to line up for the start of a race according to their anticipated pace. Unfortunately, too many slower runners line up in front of the faster runners. In addition to this not being fair, in a large race the slower participants can actually create problems by blocking the path of faster runners. In rare instances, pushing inadvertently occurs, which can lead to runners slipping and falling.

If you're not sure where to line up and are worried about whether you'll get stuck behind the slow runners or quickly left behind by the fast ones, play it safe and head for the middle of the pack. There will be runners who quickly pass you and others whom you will pass, but if you're new to running races, the middle is the best position from which to find your rhythm and enjoy the run. Take a deep breath and know that you are going to have fun, stay relaxed, and achieve your goals.

Pacing and Staying Relaxed

Running at the appropriate pace for your ability level is crucial for all distances, from sprints to the marathon, to enhance your chances of performing optimally and therefore running your fastest possible race. It is so easy to start the race running much faster than you should—and you may not even realize it! Your pace during the first mile may feel effortless due to the adrenaline rush and excitement of the event. But speed can cause you to burn out by the second or third mile.

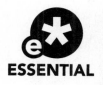

ESSENTIAL

Something you'll probably see all the runners around you doing is readying their watches prior to the start of the race. You should do the same. Be prepared so that when you hear, "Runners take your mark, set, go!" your watch is already at zero and all you have to do is push the start button to be on pace.

Be sure to check your watch at the mile markers of the race (called mile splits) to see how far off the official time you may be. The information you get from your watch as well as the split times called by the people manning the mile markers can both help you stay on pace.

For races in which many runners compete, the organization holding the event may use computer chips to time the runners. The chips activate at the starting line and stop at the finish. If you're toward the back of a pack in such a race, don't start your watch when the officials shout "Go!" (in large races, a starting pistol is fired) since it might take you a while to reach the actual starting line and your time will be thrown off. Instead, start your watch at the starting line and look at it at each mile marker. The split times shouted out by the people manning the markers may not be what you're running either because their time started when the announcer said "Go!" Working your watch this way during a big race is the only way you'll know with any sense of accuracy your true pace mile by mile, as well as your actual finish time immediately after the race.

Running each mile at the same pace is a proven approach to turning in your best race time. If you feel like you're really overextending yourself, you probably are. Taper back a bit and see whether you feel like catching some folks at the end. You'll enjoy finishing strong.

Another way to avoid draining your energy too quickly is to remember to stay loose and relaxed. Be sure to shake out your arms and shoulders occasionally throughout the race to avoid upper-body muscle tightness. This will contribute to a more comfortable run.

FACT

Chances are you'll run faster in a race than you do during your training runs, even if your goal is not to go faster. The rush of the crowd and the fact that it's a race contribute to the excitement, which usually translates into a faster pace.

Water Stops and Supplements

Most races have water stops, at which eager volunteers hold out cups of water for you to take as you pass. Mastering the art of drinking while you're running takes some practice. But the only way to do it is to, well, do it. So give it a try. If you're not too successful and get most of the water on your face or shirt, oh well. What you don't want to do is inhale the water and end up choking. So if it's easier and more comfortable for you, just slow down to a walk for a few steps while you drink.

QUESTION

What if I get injured during the race?
If you feel a significant increase in pain as you continue to run, seriously consider dropping out of the race. No race is worth the risk of hurting yourself by continuing to run and causing a minor injury to turn into a major setback.

If it's a really hot day, you can also pour water over your head, on your neck, chest, and hands. As for supplements like energy gels, you don't really need them in a 5K.

After the Race

Congratulations, you did it! Savor the excitement of finishing, no matter when you came in. Then after crossing the line, get something to drink. Within a few minutes of finishing, do a 5- to 10-minute cool-down jog to begin the recovery process. Stretch thoroughly immediately after the race. Doing so will keep muscle soreness to a minimum over the next day or two. And, of course, chat about the race with fellow runners.

When you get home, look at the flyers you collected at the race to consider when and where to run your next 5K (or maybe an even longer race). If you're like most runners, you'll be hooked on the exhilarating feeling of having successfully competed in the race.

Themed Races

Growing in popularity are novelty or theme events from which to choose that will surely add variety to one's race schedule. While a handful of runners will approach these solely for competitive purposes, fun is the emphasis for most of the participants. Organizers tend to keep the distance short, oftentimes at 5K, to attract runners of all ability and experience levels. However, some races are longer in distance: 8K (4.97 miles), 10K (6.2 miles), 12K (7.45 miles), and beyond. Many events are tied to holidays, and quite often the name of the race is a giveaway for the festive time of year being celebrated. Here's a small sampling from across the United States:

- Midnight Run 4-miler held in New York on New Year's Eve
- New Year's Day Resolution Run 5K in Seattle
- Love the Run You're With 5K held on Valentine's Day in Arlington, Virginia
- Shamrock Shuffle 8K held in Chicago on St. Patrick's Day

- Firecracker 5K held on Independence Day in Little Rock, Arkansas
- Turkey Day 5K held in Minneapolis on Thanksgiving
- Reindeer Run held the first Saturday in December in Charleston, South Carolina, to celebrate the holiday season

Speaking of holidays, Halloween isn't the only time of the year when runners get to dress in costume. A perfect example is San Francisco's Bay to Breakers 12K, where it has been a tradition since 1965 for many participants to dress in elaborate costumes or compete as part of a tethered centipede team. Clothing seems to be optional for a handful of runners, as they streak through the streets wearing as little as running shoes and race numbers! Similarly, the Stiletto Stampede is a national race series where runners, men and women alike, have the opportunity to make a fashion statement while at the same time raise awareness and support the fight against breast cancer. The rules are simple: Race 100 meters wearing stiletto heels that are at least 3 inches high!

Numerous races are associated with small-town festivals that are held in rural communities during harvest times where residents enthusiastically come out to support the runners. These events are popular for a variety of reasons: the opportunity to take a relaxed country drive, race a scenic course, and enjoy a festive atmosphere oftentimes featuring live music and crafts for sale. Best of all, everyone gets to eat the fruits, so to speak, of the harvest after the race!

For runners seeking additional challenges beyond completing the 5K distance at a fast clip to those in search of a very unique race experience, obstacle events are popping up around the country. Many are sponsored by branches of the armed services and are held at military bases. Participants run up and down slippery hills, navigate through tire obstacles and other obstructions, scale walls, crawl through tunnels and trenches, and trudge through large mud pits, all in the name of not-so-clean fun!

CHAPTER 16

Completing a 10K
and Half-Marathon

If you've come off some 5K races enjoying the experiences and are eager for the next challenge, the 10K or perhaps the half-marathon is what you should set your sights on. The 10K doubles the 5K to 6.2 miles, and just as the 5K holds sufficient challenge for every level of runner, so the 10K is also a runner-friendly distance. If you're serious about your running and taking the advice of this book, you most certainly can bring your racing distance safely up from the 5K to the 10K and from there to the half-marathon (13.1 miles) while continuing to enjoy (almost) every minute of your races.

Mileage Buildup for the 10K

Once you've run a few 5Ks and have built a consistent running base, your objective may be to run a faster 5K race the next time out. If you've yet to train for the 10K, however, your focus should be on handling the distance while running at a pace you can realistically maintain. Doing this successfully incorporates three elementals of being a runner: stamina, strength, and regulating of pace. Mastering these brings increased ability to all your runs and races.

In thinking about how to safely build your mileage to race the 10K, consult the mileage buildup schedules. There are two schedules—one for beginner and novice runners and one for advanced runners. Take a look at them to determine where you fit in based on your present running routine and your racing goals. Although both are designed to build you safely to running 10 miles, the beginner need not run more than 5 miles in training to be able to comfortably run a 10K race. On the other hand, experienced runners who have competitive aspirations for the 10K or who plan to run a longer event later in the race season may wish to build to the 10-mile level.

ESSENTIAL

Tapering consists of a gradual decrease in running. For runners who race, this means cutting back on mileage in the week before a race. What's the advantage of this? It's so that on race day your legs are rested and you can do your best.

When you follow a training schedule specific to the goal of a race, as you should when training for a significant distance like the half-marathon or marathon, you will incorporate tapering time into your schedule. For shorter distances like the 5K or even the 10K, how much to taper depends on your goals, fitness level, and current weekly mileage.

Things to Consider When Increasing Your Distance

Remember that for the 10K you want to be able to handle the distance. You need leg strength, for sure, but you also need stamina and, if it's your goal, speed. Simply coming off a 5K race in which you finished strong and felt good does not necessarily quality you for doubling that distance—at least not competitively.

To set yourself up for equally enjoyable 10Ks, keep in mind this advice:

- **Form.** As you push yourself, don't get sloppy. It's better to put in fewer miles with proper form than to overexert yourself while running in such a way that could lead to injury. Pay particular attention to staying relaxed in your upper body.
- **Pace and time.** The 10K requires a different strategy from the 5K. You need reserves to push for a strong finish after running 6.2 miles, which is quite different from running 3.1 miles. One way to gauge the effectiveness of your training program for meeting your race goal(s) is to set up some mock 10Ks. Go the distance at approximately the same time of day in similar weather conditions, taking note of when you feel the strongest, when you feel like you're starting to lag, when you get your second wind, and so on. Be sure to wear your watch on all your runs so you can become better aware of pace and determine what pace is realistic for you.
- **Energy.** Energy comes from what you eat and drink, so be sure to be smart about both.
- **Safety.** When going out on longer runs, consider in advance the time of day you're running and what the environment is like. Wear reflective gear if there will be little light; carry a cell phone; be wary of road or trail conditions; and be mindful of staying hydrated.
- **Self-talk.** If running a longer distance seems intimidating, you may find yourself nagged by unreasonable fears. Change your self-talk so that you approach your runs with positive energy and enthusiasm. If your running program is realistic and your goals are within reason, you should be able to increase your mileage fairly easily.
- **Cool down.** Run slowly the last half-mile or so of your long run to help your body ease back into your regular routine.
- **Stretch.** As discussed, a thorough stretch after a run is imperative and especially so after a long run. Stretching helps your muscles recuperate, and minimizes soreness later.

Running the 10K

When the big day finally arrives, you want to be ready. Prepare the way you would for any event, being sure to bring the gear you need with you to the race, giving yourself plenty of time to register and warm up when you get there, using the facilities if necessary (there are sometimes long lines for these!), and finding your place among the runners. Many of the same strategies and tips relating to the 5K race also pertain to the 10K.

Think about how competitive you want to be. If the race is your first 10K, you probably won't have winning as your goal. Decide on a time that you think is currently achievable for you in the race, and line up with the runners in that bracket. Posted behind the starting line at many races are signs indicating a continuum of anticipated paces that serve as a guide for runners to position themselves appropriately. It is important to place yourself based on a pace you can realistically maintain throughout the event—that is, where you won't slow others down or need to weave around those who might slow you down.

Once the race begins, settle into a pace based on your training runs for this distance. It's easy to excitedly start out too fast, especially if you feel fit and ready to tackle this new length. Rein yourself in a bit, thinking about how good you'll feel in the last few miles to have energy to draw upon in order to achieve your goal. With a quarter-mile to go, decide if you have energy reserves remaining to throw in a kick, picking up your pace all the way to the finish line.

After the 10K

Your post-race routine should be fairly standardized by now: Spend a few minutes jogging easily or walking, drinking water, and then stretching. Have a bagel, banana, or other nutritious snack. When you get home, shower, change, and you're ready for whatever your day or evening may bring!

In regard to your next race, the general formula is that for every mile raced, you should allow the same number of days before your next race. For example, if you run a 10K, then allow at least six to seven days before your next race. You'll probably feel better racing a 5K next; entering another 10K may be overdoing it. On the other hand, if you race a 5K the first weekend, doing a 10K the next could be a progressive step in your training. The success of either scenario depends on you as an individual and where you are in your training.

QUESTION

How soon after my 10K can I run a 5K?
Depending on your mileage base, experience level, and how quickly you recover coming off the 10K, you could decide to compete in a 5K over the course of the weekends that follow. Running clubs sometimes hold seasonal race series in which they stage 5K races every week over the course of six to eight weeks. These are good motivation for enjoying the experience of racing in an atmosphere of camaraderie.

Training for and Running the Half-Marathon

The desire to race a half-marathon is a natural progression for many runners who have completed a mileage buildup program and wish to meet a new goal. Although it doesn't require the same degree of commitment as training for a marathon, the half-marathon is still a worthy challenge that many runners around the world seek. It's also a practical way to gauge your endurance if you're coming off racing the 10K and want to build up to a marathon.

Mileage Buildup for the Half-Marathon

Begin your half-marathon training by finding the training week or level from one of the two mileage buildup schedules in Chapter 5 that more closely matches your present training routine. From that point, proceed until you complete the remaining mileage specified on whichever schedule you use.

Next, continue your training by following your choice of the two schedules featured next. Determine the maximum distance of your longest training run (and thus your choice of charts) based on your competitive aspirations along with how much you enjoy doing long runs. You should complete the longest training run (16 miles) no more than three weeks before the half-marathon. Run at least 12 miles in practice to be minimally prepared for the 13.1-mile race. It is important to note that while mileage is indicated in these schedules beginning two days following the half-marathon, it is crucial that you listen to your body and take additional rest days as needed to facilitate full muscle recovery.

▼ **TABLE 16-1: NOVICE HALF-MARATHON TRAINING SCHEDULE**

Week #	Sun.	Mon.	Tue.	Wed.	Thur.	Fri.	Sat.	Total
1	11	Rest	5	7	5	Rest	5	33
2	12	Rest	5	7	5	Rest	5	34
3	8	Rest	6	Rest	4	Rest	2 Optional	18–20 Taper Week
4	13.1 (race day)	Rest	4	5	4	Rest	5	31.1

Numbers refer to miles of running

▼ **ADVANCED HALF-MARATHON TRAINING SCHEDULE**

Week #	Sun.	Mon.	Tue.	Wed.	Thur.	Fri.	Sat.	Total
1	11	Rest	6	8	5	Rest	5	35
2	12	Rest	6	8	5	Rest	5	36
3	8	Rest	4	Rest	4	Rest	4	20 Easy Week
4	14	Rest	6	8	6	Rest	5	39
5	16	Rest	6	8	6	Rest	5	41
6	13	Rest	5	7	5	Rest	5	35
7	10	Rest	6	Rest	4	Rest	2 Optional	20–22 Taper Week
8	13.1 (race day)	Rest	4	6	4	Rest	4	31.1

Numbers refer to miles of running

The Long Run

While the long run is discussed in detail in the marathon training chapters of this book, the key points regarding this important workout are highlighted here. Similar to marathon training, the long run is the most important component of one's half-marathon training for teaching the body to both mentally and physically tackle the challenge of completing a race of 13.1 miles or longer. For the purpose of this discussion, the distance of a long run is considered to be 10 miles (or longer) or a run that lasts more than 90 minutes.

The long run also provides an excellent opportunity to experiment with a variety of concerns, such as shoes, nutrition, and pacing. Above all, long-distance training schedules must be designed so that runners are rested prior to undertaking their long runs. Runners who complete at least two long runs of 10–12 miles prior to a half-marathon are better prepared to face the challenge ahead of them.

ALERT

Don't split your long run! If your training schedule calls for a long run of 10 miles, you must run the distance at one time rather than splitting it into a 5-mile morning session and a 5-mile evening run.

The majority of runners who experience difficulty in completing their long training runs fail to prepare adequately for these critical workouts. The following guidelines enable you to prepare for and complete your long runs safely and successfully. Completing all your scheduled long runs in turn greatly enhances your chance of performing well on race day.

Pace and Time

Run at a conversational pace by starting out slowly to conserve glycogen. As a general guideline, particularly for runners whose primary goal is to finish the half-marathon comfortably, the pace of your long run should be approximately 1–1½ minutes slower than your present 10K race pace. You should be running so that your perceived exertion level seems easy and relaxed. Put another way, if you wished to carry on a lengthy conversation with another runner, you could easily do so without gasping for air.

There are two major reasons you need to run at a relaxed pace during the long run. Most important, you are conserving glycogen and glucose (your energy sources, converted from digested food stored in your working muscles and blood supply). Running at an easy pace also reduces the possibility of incurring an injury. This is particularly important since you are probably building your mileage to a level as yet unachieved. This in itself puts stress and strain on your muscles, joints, tendons, and ligaments.

As you focus on your pace, also consider running for cumulative time, approximating the distance you travel. For example, if your easy-run pace is 9 minutes per mile, run for 90 or so minutes for your 10-miler rather than finding a course that is exactly that distance. Doing so enables you to have more flexibility and spontaneity in regard to the route you choose to run. Schedule some long runs at the same time of day the actual race will be held to familiarize yourself with running during that time frame and also to develop a pre-race routine that feels comfortable to you.

QUESTION

Should I do long runs with others?
For your long runs, either run with friends or find a group running *at your pace*. Running with a group makes the long run more pleasurable and easier to accomplish than running alone.

Running Form and Upper-Body Considerations

Although there is no need to alter your running stride, you need to focus on keeping your upper body relaxed and loose. Remember, tension is the adversary of all long-distance runners. Tension in the arms, shoulders, and especially the back drains energy and makes running more difficult. It creates stress that detracts from the main focus—running. Shake out your arms and shoulders regularly to combat tension.

Carry your arms close to your waist or hips to conserve energy. Also avoid unnecessary armswing, particularly laterally across the body. Remember, this is wasted motion and energy expenditure, and it also puts extra strain on your hips.

Hydration

Water and sports drinks are your lifeline in completing these long runs. It is very important that you drink fluids every 25–30 minutes while you are running, regardless of weather conditions. For runs that are more than an hour long, you also need to drink sports drinks such as Gatorade®

or Powerade® to fuel those working muscles, keeping them functioning optimally.

FACT

The half-marathon is an ideal race to use as a marathon tune-up. It provides an opportunity to experiment with a variety of factors, such as pre-race routine, nutrition, and pacing. Additionally, you can to some extent extrapolate your marathon finish time from the half-marathon distance. However, marathon predictor charts have less reliability if you haven't completed at least two runs of over 20 miles.

Don't rely on your thirst mechanism to send a signal to your brain saying "I'm thirsty!" If you wait until that point, you will not be able to consume enough fluids to catch up with your hydration needs. Doing so puts you at greater risk of heat illness. In short, dehydration is one of your biggest enemies. Many beginners fail to grasp this and ignore opportunities to take in fluids. Don't pass these up. Drink!

Psychological Issues

Realize that long runs are sometimes difficult to complete and that you may experience some bad patches in the later miles. Persevering through these stretches helps you to develop mental toughness, a skill that is essential during a half-marathon or a full marathon. Use imagery, mental rehearsal or visualization, and self-talk to develop mental toughness. For example, to make the run seem more doable, try to mentally break the course into sections. That is, mentally run from one landmark to the next instead of thinking of completing the entire 10-mile training course. When you reach the first landmark, then mentally think of running to the next, and so forth.

If this seems like a real hurdle to you, review the sections on yoga and meditation. These are practices proven to help athletes stay focused and run better, with improved breathing techniques and mental acuity.

A cardinal rule of long-distance racing is: Don't try anything new or leave anything to chance on race day. Use all training runs as opportunities for experimentation.

Finally, after the run is over, continue to drink fluids (water, sports drinks, and juice are all good choices). Also eat some more; you've earned it! As soon as possible (ideally within 15 minutes of the end of the run), have something to eat to replace depleted glycogen stores. Research has shown that to avoid muscle fatigue the next day, carbohydrates should be eaten as soon as possible following long-duration exercise.

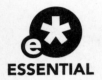

ESSENTIAL

You might want to engage in some other activities after completing your long run and half-marathon. Do some light cycling or walking later in the day to loosen up your legs. Also consider using therapeutic techniques such as dipping your legs in cool water immediately after the run or getting a leg massage over the next couple of days to reduce muscle soreness and fatigue.

Runners, Take Your Marks, Set, Race!

For the sake of discussion, assume that your half-marathon race is scheduled for Sunday at 8:00 A.M. By experimenting with concerns during your long training runs, you greatly increase the chances that your half-marathon experience will be a successful one.

First, you need to get lots of rest Saturday night. Aim for at least 8 hours of sleep. What you don't want to do is tire out your legs, so make either Friday or Saturday a complete rest day for the legs. If you must train, do something light (not a run). If you train on Saturday, make it a very light workout on the legs or, better yet, do some core work. If your friends want to go dancing, ask them to reschedule for the following week.

What to Eat and Drink

What you drink and eat can make a big difference in your performance on race day. You have to fight the possibility of dehydration, so drink water throughout the day Saturday. Remember, it is possible to drink too much water, so be careful. Additionally, you can eat a lot, but make sure you eat smart. Eat meals high in carbohydrates for lunch and dinner Saturday, but don't eat the wrong foods. Select the right pre-race meal for you, such as pasta with marinara sauce as opposed to Alfredo sauce. Avoid foods high in salt, excessive protein, and fat all day Saturday. Also, this may surprise you but go light on salads and vegetables; these can cause a host of digestive problems.

On Sunday morning, drink about 16 ounces of water prior to your race. Additionally, eat a light snack. Figure out what you must eat and how early to do so to avoid digestive problems.

While running, you want to drink lots of fluids. Be sure to stop for water frequently throughout the run. For runs and races longer than 90 minutes, you should strive to drink sports beverages every 2–3 miles or every 25–30 minutes. Drinking on the run requires careful planning of the route (make sure there is water available frequently, along with places to stash sports drinks). Most races have frequent aid stations, and almost all (with the exception of some 5Ks) provide sports drinks.

You may also want to consider using gel carbohydrate replacement products during the run for race distances longer than 10K. Be sure to chase these products down with water to avoid stomach cramps and to enhance absorption. (Please dispose of gel and energy wrappers properly by throwing them away in trash receptacles or placing them in your fanny pack. There's nothing worse than a disrespectful runner.)

Shoes, Apparel, and Accessories

You should remember that, especially for a long run, good equipment is essential. To get through the race comfortably, pay particular attention to your shoes, apparel, and accessories.

For your footwear, make sure that your shoes have low mileage to maximize absorption of shock. Do not wear new shoes or shoes that are not sufficiently broken in for a long run or race. On the other hand, make sure the shoes you wear aren't on their last legs or broken down.

In addition to shoes, comfortable and functional clothing is one of the most important ingredients for runs of all distances, particularly for long runs and races. Wear Coolmax® or synthetic-blend socks, singlets, shorts, and leggings that wick away moisture and won't cause chafing. Again, don't wear anything for the first time at the race. Wear socks and other apparel that you have worn at least once during training and that have been washed. Also remember to use Skin Lube® or Vaseline® petroleum jelly (on feet, under arms, between thighs, nipples, etc.) to eliminate or reduce chafing and/or blisters, which may bleed during a long race.

ALERT

When dressing for a run, remember that excess clothing causes over-heating of the body. Once you begin running, it will feel as if the outside temperature has risen by 10 degrees Fahrenheit. Also remember that hats trap body heat, making them perfect for a cold-weather race but a bad idea for a race with hot and humid conditions.

When the Race Is Over

You mean you have to do something after the run is over? Yes! Sometimes injuries occur as a result of not giving your fatigued muscles the cool-down they need and deserve. Follow these three simple guidelines after every long-distance run, and you'll feel better.

Drink and Eat

You've sweated the miles, burned off the calories, depleted glycogen, and torn down muscles. There will probably be food available from the race organizers when you reach the finish line. After stretching, enjoy your post-race foods, focusing on getting protein and carbs from foods like bagels, bananas, and yogurt. When you get home, you may be hungry again. Although this isn't an invitation to pig-out and throw all dietary caution to the wind, the maxims "I eat, therefore I run" and "Eat, drink, and be merry" each apply in moderation.

Cool Down

It is important to cool down once you've crossed the finish line by walking for 10–15 minutes or by jogging at least a half-mile to bring your heart rate down and to minimize muscle stiffness. It may sound crazy, but your body will in fact feel better for it.

Stretch

After you've walked or jogged a little and had something to drink, stretch thoroughly while your muscles are still warm. This can't be stated strongly enough, since your muscles will probably be tight from the long distance that you've covered. Don't wait until you've cooled off or you're more likely to hurt yourself. Also, stretching warm muscles helps make them less stiff and painful later on in the day.

CHAPTER 17

Are You Ready for the Marathon?

The marathon is one of the most grueling events in all of organized sports. It requires long months of painstaking training and planning. Finishing a marathon, however, is one of the most rewarding experiences any runner can possibly imagine. It takes dedication, resolve, and persistence. It is also something that should only be attempted by a runner who has some miles under her belt. Just as properly training to run a marathon and then completing one can be a highlight of your life, not training properly can leave you with a very bad experience and perhaps with injuries that may be difficult to overcome. If you're going to run a marathon, do it right—it's worth every minute of training.

A Brief History of the Marathon

There is probably no sporting event in the world that has more history tied to it than the marathon. It is legendary. In a nutshell, the king of the Persian Empire in the fifth century B.C. wanted to conquer Greece so he could bring his armies into Europe by land. Knowing they would be outnumbered, the Atheneans sent a foot messenger to Sparta, 150 miles away, seeking assistance to fight the Persians. That messenger was Pheidippides. He covered the distance in two days, and the Spartans were able to help the Atheneans beat back the Persian army and secure Greece. The marathon was named for the site of the battle of Marathon, approximately 25 miles from Athens, where the victory occurred.

When did the marathon become 26.2 miles? As travel writer Paul Smaras notes:

> *At the 1908 Olympic Games in London, the marathon distance was changed to 26 miles to cover the ground from Windsor Castle to White City stadium, with 385 yards added on so the race could finish in front of the royal family's viewing box. . . . After sixteen years of extremely heated discussion, this 26.2 mile distance was established at the 1924 Olympics in Paris as the official marathon distance.*

Factors to Consider When Choosing a Marathon to Enter

For many people, one of the most exciting aspects about running a marathon is traveling to a different city or region of the country. Other runners will find great comfort and enjoyment staying close to home. There are numerous factors to consider when deciding upon the marathon you wish to train for, and enter, many of these based on personal preferences. Some of these include scenery along the course (urban versus rural), size of the entry field, difficulty of the terrain, anticipated weather conditions, spectator support, and amenities provided, to name a few.

Would you rather run a marathon in a large urban center? Or would you prefer competing 26.2 miles on a rural road adjacent to mountains, trees, and streams? Would you like to be entertained along the course with bands playing every couple of miles? Or do you prefer a more solitary experience with the sounds of birds chirping or waves crashing along the beach? Do you seek the additional challenge of a course that features rolling or hilly terrain? Perhaps you find covering 26.2 miles on pancake-flat terrain demanding enough!

If this will be your first marathon, selecting an event that attracts thousands of runners and is known for great spectator support along the course can be motivating. Chances are, even in the later miles, it can be comforting to know that you will be running in the company of other runners and be cheered on by spectators, all the way to the finish line.

If your goal is to set a PR (personal record) or to qualify for the Boston Marathon, it is advantageous to seek an event held during a cool time of the year on a flat course. It can also be beneficial to select a race with a smaller entry field so you can get a fast start and are less likely to burn valuable time and energy maneuvering around other runners.

Running a marathon in your home town provides many advantages. Aside from saving hundreds of dollars on travel, lodging, and food expenses, you're likely to feel more relaxed and less stressed by sleeping in your own bed and eating home-cooked meals. Additionally, you can recruit family and friends as spectators to cheer for you along the course.

Many runners find it enjoyable to combine their marathon with vacation plans. Thus, it can be advantageous to select a race whose site is close to attractions and activities of interest, such as theme parks, beaches, or recreational areas. This is especially important if you will be traveling with family members who may not have the same enthusiasm about the marathon as you do!

It is also imperative to consider the time of year the marathon is held. If you're targeting an event held in the United States in the summer or early fall, realize that your longest runs will likely occur during hot, humid months, adding a greater level of difficulty to your training. Additionally, there is an increased chance of warmer temperatures during the race.

On a similar note, the Honolulu Marathon, which is held in early December, provides environmental challenges for runners who have completed most of their training in cooler weather but who may be unable to arrive a couple of weeks beforehand to acclimate to hot and humid conditions.

Getting Down to Business: The Long Run

You should not attempt a marathon unless you have been running for at least one year and are comfortably running 25 miles a week or more. If you find that running 25 miles per week is difficult to accomplish for any number of reasons (aches and pains, time constraints, etc.), you are not yet ready to begin training for this event.

Runners training to compete in a marathon must slowly and systematically build the distance of their long runs to a minimum of 20 miles. In fact, completing two to three runs of 20–23 miles each in the ten weeks prior to the marathon is a realistic predictor of successfully completing the race.

QUESTION

What are the benefits of the long run?
The long run strengthens the heart; it strengthens the leg muscles critical for endurance; it develops mental toughness and coping skills; it increases fat-burning capacity as well as capillary growth and myoglobin concentration in muscle fibers; and it increases aerobic efficiency.

Definition and Purposes of the Long Run

For the purpose of this discussion, the distance of a long run is 10 miles or longer (or a run that lasts over 90 minutes). As a general rule, and particularly for those whose goal is to finish comfortably, the pace of the long run should be approximately 1 minute slower than the pace at which you *realistically* expect to complete the marathon. If your training schedule calls for a long run of 18 miles, you must run the distance at one session rather than splitting it into a 9-mile morning run and a 9-mile evening run.

The long run is the most important component of marathon training because it teaches the body both to mentally and physically tackle the challenge of completing the 26.2-mile event. Physiologically, the body must learn to draw on fat-storage energy reserves after depleting glycogen fuel stores in the muscles (converted from carbohydrate food sources). You must become accustomed to running for very long periods of time. The mental toughness you develop from completing long training runs pays handsome dividends when you run the actual marathon.

Above all, design your marathon training schedule so that you are rested prior to undertaking your long runs. If you complete two to three long training runs of 20 to 23 miles, you will no doubt reduce the possibility of hitting the dreaded "wall" during the marathon. The wall refers to the point in time during a marathon when your body's glycogen stores become depleted, after which your pace can slow to a crawl.

The majority of runners who experience difficulty completing long training runs fail to prepare adequately for these critical workouts. So remember, both long runs and the marathon itself don't have to be painful experiences. The key is to plan ahead.

ALERT

It is important to follow the hard-easy method of training emphasized throughout this book. Pressing too hard without scheduled rest periods or reduced workloads more often than not leads to injuries and training delays. Do not become obsessed with your training to the extent that you run on rest days. This approach can lead to injury, fatigue, and even burnout.

Making the Long Run Easier and Safer

Don't schedule long runs too early in your training, even if you are physically prepared to cover the distance. This can lead to staleness or premature burnout. Additionally, you could peak too early in your training. Also, schedule some long runs at the same time of day the actual marathon will be held to familiarize yourself with running during that time frame and also to develop a pre-race routine you feel comfortable with.

Consider running for cumulative time, approximating the distance. Doing so gives you more flexibility and spontaneity regarding the route you will be running. However, do your longest run no closer than three to four weeks before the marathon. The distance of this run should be 23 miles *maximum*. Above all, do *not* run 26.2 miles in practice to see if you can run a marathon. Save your efforts for the actual race!

Do not increase the distance of your long run by more than approximately 10 percent over your previous long run. This equates to adding about

15–20 minutes to each subsequent long run. Every fourth week, drop the distance of your long run (along with your total weekly mileage), providing an easy week of training before the race to facilitate rest and recovery.

ALERT

When training, think about running with others whose ability level is similar to yours. Running with a group makes the long run more pleasurable and easier to accomplish than running alone. However, in running with a group, be sure you don't turn long runs into races. This will almost surely lead to injury.

Areas of Experimentation

During your marathon training you will have the opportunity to experiment with various elements that can either positively or negatively impact your marathon (for example, shoes, clothing, nutrition) prior to incorporating these practices in the actual 26.2-mile event. A cardinal rule of marathoning is: Don't try anything new on race day. Use training runs as an occasion for experimentation.

First, think about your shoes. If your shoes are causing you any discomfort during training, you should not wear them in the marathon. As soon as possible, talk to a local professional at a specialty running store for advice on a different shoe to wear for your training and racing. At least six weeks prior to the marathon, you should decide on a specific brand and model of shoe to wear for your final long training run and, of course, for the marathon.

Socks are also important. Which type of socks (for example, thin, thick, two layers, synthetic-blend) work best for you? There's no worse feeling in a marathon than developing blisters from your socks at only the halfway point!

Additionally, consider all of your running apparel. What type of clothing won't cause chafing? How much and what type of clothing do you need to wear to be comfortable yet not overheated (for example, gloves, hat, long sleeves)?

Beyond apparel, consider running accessories. For instance, do you plan to use analgesic creams (Bengay®, Myoflex®, Sportscreme®, etc.) during the marathon? Some experts claim that these don't penetrate deeply enough to relieve muscular discomfort. Others say that topical creams are effective in reducing pain and inflammation. Similarly, what about a moisturizing lubricant for your skin, such as Vaseline® petroleum jelly or Skin Lube®? If you use these products, how much and where should they be applied (for example, under arms, on toes, between thighs, on nipples)?

For your pre-race routine, consider what you are going to eat for your pre-race evening meal. What type of high-carbohydrate meal do you crave (for example, pasta, potatoes, rice)? Which foods give you the most energy? How much do you need to eat? Are there any foods that you should avoid so as not to cause digestive system problems?

Similarly, how about the race-morning snack? What type of foods work best for you, yielding energy while not causing stomach discomfort or cramps? Should you partake of caffeine? If yes, how much should you drink and how soon before the marathon? Some research suggests that drinking caffeinated products spares glycogen early in a marathon. The bottom line is that if you consume caffeine, also be sure to drink water to avoid dehydration. Another downside of using caffeine before you run is that you might end up being one of the people standing in a long line at the Porta-Potty before the race when you should be warming up!

ESSENTIAL

Many honey-makers and produce stores sell honey sticks, plastic straws filed with flavored honeys. These are very easy to carry with you on long runs since they're small and lightweight, and they provide a safe and natural source of sugar to boost your energy.

Rest is as important as eating before a race. Figure out what time you need to retire to get a good night's sleep. Also, determine how early you need to rise to take care of needs, such as eating breakfast, hydrating, and visiting the bathroom.

During the race, you need a plan for hydration. How often do you need to drink during the marathon, and should you consume sports drinks at every aid station or alternate between drinking water and sports drinks? These are very important questions you need to decide prior to your marathon.

Finally, decide whether or not you will rely on gels as a supplemental energy source during the marathon (as many runners do). There are many types of gels to choose from nowadays. The key is finding the particular product that works for you. Training runs present opportunities to decide how many packets you will need to consume during the marathon, when to take them (at which mile markers or elapsed marathon time), along with determining whether certain brands or flavors are less likely to cause stomach discomfort.

Marathon Training Schedules

Before choosing one of the two marathon training schedules that follow, it is essential that you successfully complete a base-building period by following one of the two mileage buildup schedules outlined in Chapter 5. It cannot be stressed enough that both of the marathon training schedules offered below are designed for runners who have successfully completed the mileage buildup period. If you have not fully completed the buildup phase, then *do not proceed.*

Additionally, it is crucial that you have applied the training principles and injury prevention strategies emphasized throughout this book. For example, if you ever feel excessively fatigued or are experiencing increased muscular stiffness or soreness prior to the workouts listed, it is important to make adjustments. These modifications could include reducing mileage (particularly for midweek runs) or shifting workouts to allow for an additional rest day as needed. Using a training schedule without such basic knowledge or without the consultation of a coach or the advice of a knowledgeable and experienced runner is indeed hazardous to your health.

If you cannot complete the mileage specified for the first four weeks in these schedules without injury or resultant pain, then you should continue to work through the mileage buildup schedules. Scale back your training to a level that enables you to train safely without leg fatigue, soreness, or injury.

Schedule 1 (Beginner)

Although this schedule features a bit less weekly mileage than the advanced marathon schedule that follows (Schedule 2), runners who complete the workouts specified here will still be well-prepared to run 26.2 miles successfully on marathon day. Another attractive feature of this schedule is that it is based on a four-day training week, ideal for people faced with the demands of a busy work schedule, family commitments, and other obligations and responsibilities.

▼ **TABLE 17-1: MARATHON TRAINING SCHEDULE 1 (BEGINNER)**

Week	Sun.	Mon.	Tues.	Wed.	Thur.	Fri.	Sat.	Total
1	10	Rest	5	Rest	5	Rest	4	24
2	5	Rest	4	Rest	4	Rest	4	17 Light Week
3	11	Rest	5	Rest	6	Rest	4	26
4	12	Rest	5	Rest	7	Rest	4	28
5	13	Rest	5	Rest	8	Rest	4	30
6	6	Rest	4	Rest	4	Rest	4	18 Light Week
7	15	Rest	5	Rest	8	Rest	4	32
8	17	Rest	5	Rest	8	Rest	4	34
9	19	Rest	5	Rest	8	Rest	4	36
10	7	Rest	4	Rest	4	Rest	4	19 Light Week
11	21	Rest	5	Rest	7	Rest	4	37
12	10	Rest	5	Rest	8	Rest	4	27
13	8	Rest	4	Rest	4	Rest	4	20 Light Week
14	22	Rest	5	Rest	7	Rest	4	38
15	10	Rest	5	Rest	8	Rest	4	27
16	14	Rest	5	Rest	7	Rest	4	30
17	8	Rest	6	Rest	4	Rest	Rest	18 Light Week
18	26.2 Marathon	Rest	Rest	Rest	Rest	Rest	Rest	Marathon Week

Numbers refer to miles of running (except for week numbers)

Schedule 2 (Advanced)

This is an eighteen-week program geared to the runner who has completed the more advanced mileage buildup schedule featuring higher weekly mileage. As with the beginner's marathon training schedule, you'll notice that this schedule builds up mileage gradually. In the first week you will run 34 miles total. You will gradually hit varying peaks in weeks 6, 11, and 14.

▼ TABLE 17-2: MARATHON TRAINING SCHEDULE 2 (ADVANCED)

Week #	Sun.	Mon.	Tues.	Wed.	Thur.	Fri.	Sat.	Total
1	10	Rest	6	8	6	Rest	4	34
2	12	Rest	6	8	6	Rest	4	36
3	6	Rest	4	Rest	4	Rest	4	18 Light Week
4	14	Rest	6	8	6	Rest	4	38
5	16	Rest	6	8	6	Rest	5	41
6	18	Rest	6	8	6	Rest	5	43
7	6	Rest	5	Rest	5	Rest	4	20 Light Week
8	20	Rest	5	7	6	Rest	4	42
9	14	Rest	6	8	6	Rest	4	38
10	7	Rest	5	Rest	6	Rest	4	22 Light Week
11	21	Rest	5	7	6	Rest	4	43
12	14	Rest	6	8	6	Rest	4	38
13	8	Rest	6	Rest	6	Rest	4	24 Light Week
14	22–23	Rest	5	7	6	Rest	5	45–46
15	12	Rest	6	8	6	Rest	4	36
16	14	Rest	5	Rest	7	Rest	4	30
17	10	Rest	6	Rest	4	Rest	1–2 Optional	21–22 Taper Week
18	26.2 Marathon	Rest	Rest	Rest	Rest	Rest	Rest	Marathon Week

Numbers refer to miles of running (except for week numbers)

Mentally Training for the Marathon

This section discusses a variety of mental training strategies for the marathon. These enable you to set realistic goals, complete the necessary physical training (in particular, the long runs), and be prepared mentally for the challenges ahead.

FACT

Techniques you can use to psyche yourself up during both marathon training and the actual race include mental rehearsal or visualization (creating scenarios in your mind), guided imagery (imagining how you wish an event to occur), and self-talk (giving yourself positive affirmations).

Before You Begin

There are certain mental characteristics that a runner must possess in order to undertake the necessary training that a marathon requires. These include motivation, self-discipline, and effective time-management, all of which are interrelated. Although a coach can evoke interest and enthusiasm in a training program, you must develop motivation and discipline primarily within yourself.

Set Your Goals

In order to run a marathon, you need two overarching goals to motivate and sustain you. These divide into process goals and outcome goals.

Process goals focus on mastering a task and increasing your skill level. Examples of process goals include following a training schedule as closely as possible; improving your nutrition; reading as much as you can about training principles; consulting with your coach regularly; getting increased sleep to be as rested as possible; maintaining your running journal; and making sure you replace your shoes before they become too worn.

Outcome goals relate to the finished product or, stated differently, goals you hope to accomplish in the marathon. Examples include breaking 4 hours; running the second half of the marathon faster than the first 13.1 miles; defeating a rival; and running a personal best.

There are factors to take into consideration in order to create meaningful goals for yourself in a marathon. These include:

- **Timing (present life situation).** Be sure that this is a good time in your life to pursue a marathon goal. For example, if you are relocating to take a job in another city, it might be best to wait until you settle in before training for a marathon.
- **Training information.** Take a look at two or three additional sources of credible training information to understand the commitment (of time and effort) needed to achieve your marathon goal. Books, magazine articles, and Internet sites feature a variety of marathon training programs.
- **Enjoy the journey.** First and foremost, make sure your marathon goal is something you enjoy working toward and accomplishing. If you are contemplating training for a marathon but don't enjoy running more than 30 minutes at a time, you won't enjoy training for 2–3 hours at a time over the course of many weekends.
- **Enjoy the destination.** Is the outcome of your marathon goal something you would enjoy? Is the payoff worth your time and effort? Running for a charitable cause, fulfilling a life dream and earning a medal, or traveling to a beautiful destination to run a marathon with friends can be powerful motivators to see your goal through to completion.
- **Necessary weekly training time.** Be sure that you have adequate time to train during the course of the week, taking into consideration your personal and professional obligations. Be aware of the training time commitment necessary to achieve your marathon goal.
- **Necessary long-term training time.** Prior to setting a marathon goal, be sure you have adequate time to build mileage safely and consistently based on the date of the race. Look at the miles or minutes you are currently running when considering the feasibility of running a marathon.
- **Natural ability.** Unfortunately, not everyone is born to develop into a world-class athlete. Improvement comes quickly and relatively easily in the beginning of training, but progress doesn't come nearly as rapidly after months and years of hard work. The natural ability you are born with plays a significant role in determining your marathon outcome.

- **Be sure the goal is yours.** Just because Joe down the street is training for a marathon and has urged you to join him doesn't mean you should send off your application, too. In other words, don't get swept up emotionally and commit to a marathon goal without thinking it through.
- **Establish short-term goals leading to the big goal.** If you wish to run a marathon six months from now, then set some short-term goals along the way such as entering a 10K or half-marathon to keep motivated. Although it's okay to think about where you want to be years from now, focus on realizing short-term goals within a period of six months. At the same time, you can't train hard for more than three or four months at a time. Allow breaks after attaining short-term goals or peak events during your training.
- **Congruence of activities.** To reduce your chances of incurring injury, be sure the cross-training activities you undertake are in service to your marathon goal rather than a drain. For marathon training, which requires building your long run and weekly mileage, it is wise to give up stop-and-go sports (basketball, soccer) and lateral sports such as tennis until you complete your marathon.
- **Congruence of goals.** Understand that the training necessary to run a fast mile is quite different from that for running a marathon. If you want to include some short-distance races in your marathon training schedule, plan your long run sequences so as not to miss these important workouts.

Make sure your marathon goals are realistic and reflect varying levels of difficulty, with even the most challenging goal attainable for you.

ALERT

When setting goals, it is best to be as specific as possible. Be sure to write your goals down, not only in your running journal but, say, on an index card left in a visible place, like on your refrigerator. This practical strategy will help you to achieve both short- and long-term marathon goals.

Finding someone to guide and encourage your training can be a great help. If possible, find a coach with a reputation both for enthusiasm and a positive attitude. Such traits can inspire and motivate you. Or join a group whose members share your marathon goals and can provide needed emotional support. It is essential to find fellow runners who run at your approximate pace so that your long runs do not turn into races.

Mental Strategies

Realize that marathon training is not always easy. If running a marathon were simple, there would be no challenge and everyone could do it. To enable you to cope with the physical and mental demands of completing the long training runs and running the actual marathon, particularly when the going gets tough, there are several mental strategies you can adopt. Here are mental preparation tools for meeting the difficulties of the long run.

Self-Talk

Talking to yourself, figuratively speaking of course, is an easy yet very effective way of keeping yourself on track. Here are phrases you might try keeping in the forefront of your mind:

- "If this were easy, then everybody could complete a marathon."
- "If I quit now, I'll be very disappointed in myself later this afternoon."
- "I'm not really physically tired; I'm more mentally fatigued."
- "In just one more hour this run will be finished, and I'll be at home showering, relaxing, eating."

Imagery and Visualization

Imagine a situation in which you succeed at doing something, and it can become a reality. For example, imagine yourself as a world-class marathoner running in the lead of the Boston Marathon. Imagine that your running form is smooth and graceful. Imagine that you are running effortlessly and very relaxed. You'd be surprised at how much this technique can help you.

Visualization is a vivid way to envision yourself accomplishing your marathon goal. Try these visualizations: Picture yourself running each and every mile of the marathon you are training for. Visualize the finish line with a clock displaying the elapsed time you're shooting for. See in your mind's eye all the spectators cheering for you. Think of all your friends back home pulling for you while you are running.

The Week Before the Marathon

Tapering is a process you'll begin two weeks before a race. You'll notice in the marathon training schedules that Week 17 is the taper week. The idea is to slow down. Less is best! Give your body the rest it needs to prepare for the big event. Do not use this time to fit in extra exercise in hopes of burning calories to knock off a few pounds. Your body needs to be loose and rested.

Keep stretching as much as possible over the couple of weeks prior to the marathon. Consider getting a leg massage no later than two days before the marathon—although if you've never had a leg massage, don't try it now. Take care of long toenails, blisters, and calluses the week or two prior to the marathon.

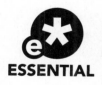

ESSENTIAL

While you're running the race, take time to enjoy the spectators, your fellow runners, and the scenery of the course. Stop negative thoughts dead in their tracks, and change them to positive affirmations. Think about how proud family members and friends will be of you.

As you taper your running, concentrate on reading books and magazine articles that provide you with motivation and inspiration. Take care of any anxieties and mental concerns in the weeks prior to the marathon. Preparation is the best strategy to reduce or eliminate stress and anxiety, which is all the more reason to have completed those key long runs in the weeks prior to the marathon. Similarly, getting a head start on packing if you are traveling out of town for the race is another way to reduce your stress level.

Remember that it is normal to be tense or nervous prior to your running a marathon. Even the most seasoned runners experience these feelings. Stay away from participants who are excessively stressed out or negative so they don't adversely affect your state of mind.

Think about Food

As you scale back the distance and intensity of your running during the last week, realize that you are not burning as many calories. Weight gain the week before a race is due to glycogen accumulation, and you should expect this. However, this does not mean to go on a crash diet! Exercise care in selecting foods to eat during this time period, aiming for nutritionally rich foods rather than simple carbs and high-fat products.

Make sure you consume plenty of carbohydrated foods three days before the marathon. Choose foods for lunch and dinner that are high in carbohydrates (such as pasta, potatoes, and rice). Don't neglect fruits, vegetables, and some protein sources. Try to really scale back on fats during this time.

Hydrate well the week before the marathon (water is best) and, in particular, during the carbohydrate-loading period three days prior to the marathon. Research shows that carbohydrates convert to glycogen more effectively when consumed with water. If you do gain a couple of pounds, don't worry about it; these glycogen reserves will serve as fuel during the marathon.

If you are traveling out of town, be sure to pack healthy snack foods to eat the weekend before the marathon. Eliminate the need to search for a grocery store that stocks your favorite foods. If traveling by plane to your marathon destination, check with your airline to see whether you're allowed to carry bottled water with you. If you can't bring your own on board, be sure to let the flight attendant know you'll need several refills while you're in the air. Flying at high altitudes causes dehydration.

CHAPTER 18

The Marathon Experience

The previous chapter discussed how to train for running the marathon up to the final days. This chapter focuses on the final preparations in the final day or two before and on running the marathon itself. This includes racing strategy and injury precautions as well as what to expect and what to do when the marathon is over. Finally, this chapter exposes you to the next level of running: ultra-running.

Physical Preparation

After training so intensely for so long, you're going to feel like you're sabotaging everything by not continuing to work hard the week before the marathon. But listen up: *Don't!* Stick to your schedule and taper as indicated.

This doesn't mean you should be completely inactive or overeat the week before the race. It's a good idea to stretch as much as possible, always remembering first to warm up your muscles through exercise. In the week prior to the race, take some brisk walks or do some light cycling. Don't do any activity that's going to strain your legs—just something to keep the blood flowing and endorphins up.

On a similar note, if you are traveling to an exciting destination for your marathon and planning on doing some sightseeing by foot, do so no later than two days prior to the race. In fact, if your time is more limited, refrain from taking any long walks the day prior to the marathon. Instead, do your sightseeing from the window of a tour bus or car to conserve your energy for the race.

Packing for an Out-of-Town Marathon

For out-of-town events in particular, don't wait until the night before you travel to collect and pack needed items. Rather, make a list of things you wish to take and begin gathering them in the days prior to departure. Also, pin your race number in advance to the front of your singlet or T-shirt. It's a good idea to take some toilet paper with you to the race site in case there's none remaining when you visit the restrooms.

A day or two before the race, check the weather forecast for the marathon site. Plan and pack for all possible types of weather conditions, given the season. Even if your online weather forecaster predicts great weather for marathon day, conditions can change. Although you can't control the weather, you can prepare for it. Don't worry about overpacking; it's better to have everything you need than to have to buy articles at the last minute in perhaps an unfamiliar place.

The Essentials

If you're flying to an out-of-town race, pack your running shoes and essential marathon apparel in carry-on luggage in case your baggage should be lost or delayed. Due to variables such as weather conditions and food preference, the following essentials list is suggestive. Try to allow for all contingencies.

- **Clothing:** Singlet,* shorts,* sports bra,* socks,* shoes,* gloves,** hat,** T-shirt (long and short sleeve),** sweatshirt,** tights,** warm-ups (jacket and long pants)**
- **Other handy items:** Running watch, Vaseline® petroleum jelly, Skin Lube® or BodyGlide®, foot powder, handkerchief, shoe laces, small gym bag, lock for locker, towel, race confirmation (to receive race number, if applicable), ibuprofen (or other pain and anti-inflammatory medicine), safety pins, sweat bands, analgesic creams (for example, Bengay®, Myoflex®).
- **Possible food items***: PowerBars®, gel supplements (for example, GU Energy Gel®, Clif Shots®, PowerBar Gel®), snack items (such as bagels, whole-grain muffins, honey sticks, fruit), carbo-loaded sports drinks, bottled water. (Since airlines no longer allow you to bring bottled liquids on board, if you are flying, plan on purchasing water at your final destination.)

[NOTE]*If traveling to the race by air, pack these in carry-on luggage in case your checked bag does not arrive with you.

**Optional items to wear prior to and/or during the marathon. (Consider bringing clothing you can discard during the race after you warm up.)

***Be sure that you have experimented with all food items comprising your pre-race diet.

What about a Cell Phone?

This is a question only you can answer for yourself. Certainly, carrying cell phones everywhere has become part and parcel of the way we live today, so that not having one on you can feel strange. A phone can just as easily clip on your running shorts or leggings as on the waistband of your everyday jeans, or you can carry the phone in a small fanny pack while you run. For long runs and marathons, it's important that the pack you use to carry the phone doesn't chafe or bump against you. Reasons you might want a cell phone on you are:

- **Emergency.** Hey, accidents happen, and despite your careful planning and preparation, misfortune could come your way on race day. If you must stop running for some reason during the marathon, there will be assistance on the course, but having a phone would surely come in handy.
- **Child care.** The time commitment you make to a marathon spans many hours. If you leave children in someone else's care, you may want the caretaker to reach you in an emergency situation.
- **To find someone.** Even if you specify a time and place to meet up with family or friends after the race, circumstances might change. A quick call or text message can save anxious waiting time for everyone involved.

Even with such compelling reasons to have a cell with you, remember that many thousands of people, in fact, the vast majority, have run and continue to run marathons without cell phones.

Other Travel Considerations

No matter how far you're traveling to the marathon, make sure you arrive in plenty of time. Allow for possible airline or traffic delays so you don't feel rushed. If you're traveling to another time zone, particularly one with a time difference of more than 1 hour, give yourself time to arrive and acclimate.

The same holds if you'll be running in an environment significantly different from the one you're used to training in. For example, if you live in Maine and you're running a December marathon in Hawaii, try to arrive there at least a week prior to the race to acclimate as much as possible to the higher temperature and humidity you'll experience during the race. Acclimating to heat and humidity takes a minimum of a week.

Know Where You're Going

Try to find a hotel close to the start and finish of the race. If they're all beyond your budget, are already booked, or you want to stay with a friend or family member in the area, map out how you're going to get to the race start in plenty of time. Better yet, drive to the start location the day before to make sure you know the best roads to get there and where you will park. Oftentimes, roads near the course are closed the day of the marathon, thus limiting your access to the start of the race.

Be sure to carefully read all official marathon literature prior to the event to familiarize yourself with procedures (documentation you need to obtain your race number, such as a photo ID, road closures, start and finish line procedures, location of aid stations and portable toilets, and shuttle bus schedules, to name just a few). Don't assume the marathon starting line will be set up adjacent to the site of race headquarters on the day prior (where registration and an exposition is often held), or you will be in for a big shock.

The Final Hours Before the Marathon

The night before and the morning of the race, you might be nervous enough that you probably won't want to socialize much, even with your family. You'll want to retire early the night before, taking your mind off the race until the next morning. Ensuring your peace of mind may necessitate spending the money for the convenience of a hotel located near the start of the race. (Plan to stay with friends or family the night following the race, when you'll want to celebrate.)

Be sure to eat proven carbohydrate products during your carbo-loading period. Keep pasta sauces simple, avoiding high-fat varieties (for example, Alfredo and pesto). Avoid eating salad and vegetables (roughage), which may prove troublesome on race day by causing digestive system problems. Stick to water before, during, and after the evening meal. Avoid coffee and tea the night before the race since they may make it difficult for you to fall asleep easily.

Rest and Relax

After your evening meal, try not to think about the marathon any more that evening. Instead, watch television, read (about something other than running), or find something restful to do until turning in for the evening.

Prior to retiring, set two alarm systems to wake you up (alarm clock, wake-up call, running-watch alarm setting, cell phone—whatever works).

Although this precaution may seem compulsive, the key is to not leave over-sleeping to chance.

Wake up early enough so as not to feel rushed. The few hours before the marathon is a time to relax yet stay focused as much as possible.

The Pre-Race Morning

Here's a checklist for the morning of your race:

- Wake up early enough to take care of everything you must do (eat and drink, visit the bathroom, dress, and so on).
- If you haven't already done so, formulate a plan to meet your family members or friends at a designated time and place after the race. Have a backup plan if for some reason you are unable to meet at a predetermined time and location after the race.
- Check the weather forecast again for updated information about conditions, temperature range, and wind. Obtaining this information helps in deciding what to wear for most of the marathon. Above all, don't overdress.
- Finally, leave for the race site from your lodging or home with plenty of time to spare, arriving early enough to check any bag and take care of last-minute details. Stay off your feet as much as possible prior to the race. Continue to drink fluids up to 15 minutes before the start of the race. Eat your final snack no later than 30 minutes before the start of the race.

During the Marathon

Runners will start lining up about 15 minutes or more before the starting time, depending on how big the participant field is. Line up according to your expected pace (faster runners to the front). In a large race the slower runners can actually create problems by blocking the path of faster runners. In rare instances, pushing inadvertently occurs which can lead to runners stumbling and falling. Please be courteous!

Also, don't get too caught up in the hoopla by being overly exuberant, yelling, and cheering as the gun is about to go off. Save that energy for later when you'll need it. Instead, focus on positive thinking. Visualize all your friends pulling for you and all the hard training you've done for this big race. Take a deep breath, and know that you are going to not only finish the race but also achieve your marathon goals.

Pacing

Running at the correct pace for your ability level is crucial in the marathon, especially for the first-time marathoner. It is so easy to start the race running much faster than you have planned or should do. But if you start out too fast, you'll pay dearly for the mistake in the later miles of the race.

A much better strategy is to start out slower than the speed you hope to average and then run the middle miles at your chosen (hopefully realistic) pace. It's a better strategy to pick up the pace during the final miles when you know you can finish rather than starting aggressively and hanging on for dear life toward the end. In the world of marathoning, there's no principle of banking the fast miles early in the race and then holding on in the end. If you go that route, you will most assuredly visit the dreaded "wall."

Take into consideration weather conditions and course difficulty in predicting your marathon time. Strong winds, high temperatures, driving rains, and hills can add several minutes to your finish time. During the marathon, constantly monitor how you are feeling, and adjust your pace accordingly based on your perceived energy level. Your previous long training runs will provide you with the experience to pace yourself.

Aid Stations

Do not pass up any fluid station. While it's okay to drink water only in the early miles, marathoners must consume sports beverages no later than 60 minutes after beginning to run. Find out through advance practice runs what works best for you.

Water is usually offered at the first tables of an aid station and sports beverages served near the end of the station. If you're not sure whether water or sports drink is in the cup, politely ask. It's not a good feeling splashing what you think is water on your head or chest to cool off and discovering a second or two later that the cool liquid is actually a sports drink!

Here's a proven method for drinking while running through the aid stations: Squeeze the top of the paper cup into a *V* shape to ensure a smooth delivery of fluid directly into your mouth. If you haven't mastered the fine art of drinking on the run (or prefer not to), it's perfectly fine to walk through the aid stations in order to consume the entire contents of the cup.

Supplementing

Many runners are taking advantage of the wide variety of energy gel products available to endurance athletes. These provide a fairly quick source of carbohydrate energy. Be sure you chase them down with water to avoid stomach cramps and to ensure absorption.

Some runners stop and eat a PowerBar®, orange slices, jelly beans, etc., to consume the calories they need. You don't want to possibly sabotage your race by ingesting something at an unofficial station of questionable freshness or quality. Experiment during your long runs with any food products you plan to eat during the marathon, and if they're light enough, think about carrying them in a non-chafing fanny pack. Or consider asking a friend or family member to hand you food at a certain point along the course.

Socializing

Chances are good you will encounter other runners running at your pace during the marathon who engage you in conversation. Whether you wish to stick with them and chat along the way is a personal decision. The positive aspect of socializing is that many great friendships have started this way, and that it can be a good way to take your mind off the physical discomfort you may face later in the marathon. Mutual pacts are often made to provide motivation for each runner to finish.

Another view is that talking might rob you of valuable energy you'll need later. The last miles of the marathon can be quite draining mentally. For that reason alone, you may choose to run the last miles without much conversation. Also, running with someone may slow you down. You'll undoubtedly finish the marathon, but sticking with someone who is slower could compromise your chance of achieving a time goal you've set for yourself.

Don't feel you need to be overly sociable at the price of losing sight of your marathon goals. If you really hit it off with someone, ask for her name and then see if you can arrange to meet after the race to share race stories while enjoying refreshments. A fellow competitor should understand your training investment and accommodate your goal, even if it means being left behind at some point. You certainly don't want to reach the finish knowing in your heart and soul that you could have done better. Don't cheat yourself.

On the Course

Once the race is underway, think pacing and overall goals. Remember what you set out to do and monitor yourself so you have the greatest chance to succeed. You will no doubt be buoyed by the energy of the runners around you and of the spectators along the course. Tap into it and let it carry you along, but don't get overzealous and run too fast at first.

Here's where reinforcing self-talk can come in handy, too. Turn your focus inward and remind yourself why you're running. Congratulate yourself for being in the marathon, for realizing your goals, and for being in good health.

ALERT

If you feel an increase in pain as you continue to run, seriously consider dropping out of the marathon. No race is worth the risk of causing a minor injury to turn into a major setback.

For example, a first-time marathoner reminded herself at every mile marker along the way of two different things she was grateful for. Reminding herself of her many blessings became an ongoing way of staying motivated and positive. If you think it might be difficult to come up with fifty-two things (plus a few more when you cross the finish line!), think again—or re-examine your life. Doesn't it feel good to be alive, good to be in an actual race, geared up to run 26.2 miles? Relish the journey!

If you've never run a marathon, there is no way to fully understand in advance the special feelings you will experience during the event. Savor and enjoy each and every moment. Take in all the sights and sounds along the way. High-five the extended hand of a child who views you as an athlete competing at center court. Smile at the spectator who tells you, "You're looking strong." Offer some brief words of encouragement to a fellow runner who may not be feeling as strong as you are. Enjoy the diverse scenery along the race course, whether from a bridge you cross, a hill affording a panoramic view of the countryside, or at the sight of storefronts while you cruise down Main Street. Along with the accomplishment of a goal you've worked so hard to achieve, you will be creating memories.

After the Marathon

Right after you finish running, do the following:

- After crossing the line and turning in either the stub on your race number, your index card, or computer chip (each marathon has its own finish-line record-keeping system), the first thing you need to do is to get something to drink and eat.
- Determine whether you need to visit the medical tent. Blisters and excessive pain in muscles and joints should be checked out by the medical personnel on hand.
- Within a few minutes of finishing, grab something to eat and again drink.
- Stretch thoroughly within 20 minutes of finishing.
- Do not even consider lying down: Keep walking.
- Sign up for a post-race massage (if available).

After you return home or to your hotel, have a nice lunch. This should be a well-balanced meal that includes the majority of calories in carbohydrates. Don't overlook consuming at least 25 percent of total calories from protein sources.

Do not take a nap or lie down for long periods of time (that is, unless you wish to be very sore or nauseous). Instead, stay on your feet by taking a walk or perhaps going for an easy bike ride of a few miles. Above all, keep moving to minimize leg muscle soreness.

Later that afternoon or evening, go out and celebrate. If you trained properly and followed all of the pre-race and marathon strategies, you should be able to do just about anything you wish (including dancing!). Above all, have a great time.

Post-Marathon Evaluation

The marathon is a mystical event because so many factors come into play in determining how well you do and how much discomfort you will experience. With the marathon behind you, it's now time to think about practices you did correctly along with errors you may have made in your training and racing. Following are evaluation questions to consider in assessing your total marathon experience, both training for and participating in the race. If necessary, modify and adjust your program to address these issues the next time you train for a marathon.

It's important to reflect upon what you might have done better or differently if you had had the chance. If you have any desire to run another marathon (which many runners do), you'll want to make the next one easier and more successful than the one you've just completed.

Marathon Report Card Checklist

You should review your overall experience by considering the following: Did you train smart and make it to the starting line healthy and injury-free? Did you avoid injury throughout your training, enabling you to complete most of your scheduled workouts? Did you listen to your body and make minor adjustments to your training schedule, thus becoming stronger and not worn down?

Think also about how your training contributed to your marathon performance. Did you train consistently? Did you complete most of the training runs (even the 18- to 23-milers)?

Evaluate your race strategy. Did you eat and drink properly before, during, and after the marathon (and the long training runs)? Did you run at the correct pace for your present ability and conditioning level during the marathon (and the long training runs)? Did you make adjustments for unforeseen problems (for example, blisters, chafing, stomach discomfort, muscle cramps) during the marathon (and the long training runs)?

Finally, think about your mental approach to the marathon. Did you have the best possible psychological attitude during the marathon (and throughout your training)? Were your marathon goals realistic?

Staying Motivated and Combating Burnout

It is not uncommon for runners to experience varying degrees of post-event depression (the blahs, decreased motivation, etc.) after finishing a marathon. This is due in part to achieving a goal that took a lot of time and energy. Now that you have accomplished the goal, you might feel a void in your life. Until you are ready both mentally and physically to set new goals, consider the following strategies to deal with reduced motivation and/or burnout: Run simply for fun, not worrying about following a training schedule; supplement your running by participating in cross-training activities; take a break from running altogether; spend more time with family and friends, and enjoy more social activities or nonathletic hobbies.

Life After the Marathon

After experiencing the personal satisfaction of completing their first marathon, many runners are interested in returning to their training immediately. Although completing a marathon is quite exciting and therefore motivating, you must take extreme care in the weeks and months following the event to rebuild mileage to pre-marathon levels. The effects on your musculoskeletal system are significant, for your muscles have undergone microtrauma (small tears of the muscle tissue that normally occur as a result of the physical demands of the marathon). These muscular tears require adequate time to properly heal. Jumping right into a heavy training schedule slows down the recovery of muscles and soft connective tissue.

Even if microtrauma damage to your muscles is minimal, your joints, bones, and other soft tissue are in a vulnerable state for days or weeks following the marathon. To reduce the possibility of an injury, you should take a prudent approach to the full resumption of training.

Some experts argue that runners should take a couple of weeks off with no running after a marathon. However, it is the recommendation of this book that you engage in cross-training activities to maintain cardiovascular fitness, while at the same time allowing your body to heal. Listen to your body and don't push it! If your body tells you that it needs more time to recover, by all means give it the rest that it needs.

Reverse Taper

You should view the next four to six weeks as a reverse taper. It is better to not run at all during the first week following the marathon than it is to jog lightly. Do some light runs the second week and build your running back over the subsequent weeks. Eat healthy. A high-carbohydrate diet in the first few days after the marathon will help replenish your depleted carbs, and protein will help to rebuild damaged muscle tissue.

With plenty of sleep and some easy walks, you'll be ready to run again in no time. Remember that the basic recovery process takes about a month, during which time you should continue to rest, run easy, avoid speed work, and keep your carbohydrate load high. The rule of taking one day of recovery for each mile raced is a rule you should seriously follow. Make sure you take the time to properly recover. If you are having serious pain (more than the usual post-marathon aches and pains), you should plan to visit a sports medicine specialist.

Scheduling Your Next Marathon

Even if you have performed well in one marathon, be careful not to race too soon because you are at a high risk for injury during the next six to eight weeks. Running another marathon, a fast 10K or 10-miler, or deciding to do another 20-mile training run, say, between marathons that are spaced too close together could be enough to cause a lingering injury.

So how long should you wait before running? The answer to that question depends on many factors. These include (but are not limited to): your years of running experience; the type and intensity of the training program you've followed with your last marathon; the energy and effort you expended during that marathon; and the duration and completeness of leg recovery after your last marathon.

Most experts say that two marathons are the limit you should run per year (spaced six months apart). The central consideration is that the body needs adequate time to recover from a marathon. Training for and competing in another marathon before your legs have fully recovered can lead to a variety of overuse injuries and staleness.

What's Next: Ultra-Running

As if running 26.2 miles weren't quite far enough, ultra-marathoning is becoming increasingly popular. The shortest standard ultra-marathon race is 50K (31 miles), making it a distance within reach for those who have conquered the marathon and are seeking a new challenge. Other common ultra-marathon events are 50-milers, 100K (62 miles), or 100 miles long. However, the distance of some races are well beyond 100 miles, and there are also 24-hour and even longer duration running events.

If after you have run two or three marathons you feel like attempting an ultra-marathon, it is recommended that you do as much research as possible before training for this next step. Research ultra-running and ultra-marathoning websites, read running magazines, gather information, and talk to specialists for advice. Whether you work with a coach or an experienced ultra-runner, you should try to find someone who can competently guide you to this next level. To put it mildly, the world of ultra-running is not for everybody. Exercise caution and prudence when attempting something of this magnitude.

FACT

There are two magazines that are ultra-running's standard bearers. They are *Marathon & Beyond* (*www.marathonandbeyond.com*) and *Ultrarunning* (*www.ultrarunning.com*). One of the best ultra-marathon websites is Kevin Sayers's "UltRunR" (*www.ultrunr.com*). Another good website is "Extreme Ultrarunning" at *www.extremeultrarunning.com*.

The world of ultra-runners is highly organized through international governing bodies, national organizations, and many clubs. The American Ultrarunning Association (AUA) is the United States branch of the

International Association of Ultrarunners (IAU). These organizations develop the rules and policies that most of the popular and legitimate events abide by. The AUA is also a member of USA Track & Field (USATF). Contact the American Ultrarunning Association (*www.americanultra.org*) to find the club nearest you.

Ultra-Running Events

The events comprising ultra-running vary greatly. The types of races and the way winners are determined are not always the same from race to race. The winners of some of the shorter ultra-marathons, such as the 50-mile races, are determined just like the popular distance races, from the mile race to the marathon: First to cross the finish line wins.

FACT

In the ultra-marathoning world, a series of races known as the Grand Slam of Ultrarunning is the most renowned. The big four races, run in the same year, that comprise the Grand Slam are: The Western States Endurance Run (100 Miles), the Vermont 100 Endurance Run, the Leadville Trail 100, and the Wasatch Front 100 Mile Endurance Run. If you complete all of these events in a year, as many ultra-marathoners aspire to do, you would log a total of 400 miles!

The other type is a fixed-time event. The parameter is given, such as 24 hours, 48 hours, or 6 days. The runner who runs the most miles within that time period wins. There are also point-to-point events.

Ultimately, there are no rules in ultra-running. You can stop to eat, rest, walk, and even sleep. It's fairly free and easy. The only penalty is that you are losing time doing these things while your competitors are running.

Training for Ultra-Runs

The training for an ultra-marathon goes way beyond what is described in this book. However, many of the same running principles apply. For example, you cannot jump from here to there. Building mileage slowly and systematically is the key to preparing properly while reducing the likelihood of injury. Stretching is still important.

Physical Preparation

How do ultra-runners cover these long distances, both in training and during the actual events? The evolution of Jeff Galloway's famous Run-Walk-Run™ marathon training method (*www.jeffgalloway.com*) can perhaps be traced to the cornerstone of ultra-training, which consists of interspersing running with frequent walking breaks.

The specific ratio of walking to running varies depending largely on the experience and ability level of the ultra-runner. Some throw in a 2-minute walking break for every mile run. Others may find that walking 3 minutes for every 10 minutes running enables them to cover increasingly longer distances.

For this strategy to be effective, you must implement walking breaks at the beginning of the run or race, not when your leg muscles are at the point of fatigue or breakdown. In short, regularly scheduled walking breaks greatly increase the ultra-runner's range, in comparison with running the entire training or racing distance. Including frequent walking also reduces the wear and tear on the leg muscles, a critical injury-prevention strategy.

ALERT

Psychologically, the ultra-marathon requires new adjustments. One of the challenges is finding ways to pass hours and hours of time mentally. Ultra-runners comment that there is no limit to the variety of topics they think about while running, ranging from the practical and conventional to the absurd!

More competitive ultra-runners integrate advanced training techniques emphasizing strength and endurance into their training schedules. These include speed workouts focusing on longer repeat interval distances (fast-paced running for 800 meters and longer) as well as the inclusion of hill training. In short, their workouts are quite different from that of those racing much shorter distances, such as the 5K or 10K, although they follow the same advanced training guidelines and precautions. However, ultra-runners practice speed work and hill training as discussed in earlier chapters. Nutrition is still paramount. Weight training is still important. And coaches in the sport still caution their runners not to overtrain, if that seems possible in preparing for such events.

Other Preparations

Nutritionally, ultra-marathoners eat greater quantities, and they eat more frequently during their events than marathoners. Their training schedules tend to be made up of more long runs than in those of marathoners. Because the weather conditions during these extra-long events can change drastically (due to topographical variations of the course along with the range from morning to night), ultra-runners must be prepared to add or strip multiple layers of clothing at a moment's notice. The same changeability can be said about terrain. One minute these athletes are running through the desert, and an hour later they may be climbing a mountain. An ultra-runner has to be thoroughly prepared for competing in such an event.

CHAPTER 19

Girls (Women!) Just Want to Have Fun

Everyone knows the adage that men and women are different. In the world of running, women and men differ as well—though both sexes have achieved incredible results. Are the differences profound or significant enough for women to have an entire section of this book dedicated to them? The answer is a resounding "Yes!"

Comparing Men and Women Runners

Before detailing significant differences, it's important to point out that there are many similarities between men and women runners. First, the biomechanics of running does not differ between men and women. Posture and stride affect the results of males and females in the same way. Neither do training techniques vary from men to women. Both men and women can and should follow the various training schedules provided in this book. With little or no variation, both men and women can do the speed workouts, cross-training, weight training, and stretching discussed in previous chapters. Additionally, men and women routinely run in the same races.

FACT

Amazingly, it wasn't until 1900 that women's events were included in the Olympic Games, and it wasn't until 1928 that women's track and field was added. In that year, American Betty Robinson won a gold medal in the 100-meter race.

In any of these areas, little separates the two sexes. However, there are also numerous factors that are specific to the female runner. Let's cover a few of the differences here.

Body Type

Women runners genetically carry more body fat than men—approximately 5–10 percent more. Men tend to have larger hearts and lungs, which deliver oxygenated blood faster and in greater quantity than those of their female counterparts. This allows muscles to respond better and faster. Men also tend to have greater muscle mass and stronger bones.

This is not to say that there aren't women runners who finish ahead of men in a lot of races. However, these biological differences explain why elite male runners are nearly always faster than accomplished women of track and field. This is particularly true in sprinting. However, the gap in performance between elite-caliber men and women narrows as race distances become longer. This is especially so in race distances of the marathon and longer.

Menstruation

Just because the discomforts of monthly menstruation are common-place for women doesn't mean they go unnoticed. Menstrual side effects (bloating, cramps, mood swings) can affect women's very participation and performance in both training and racing. At certain times, heavy menstrual flow and/or severe cramps may keep some women from exercising at all.

Although the prospect of strapping on a pair of running shoes and shorts and hitting the pavement may not seem appealing to women during men-struation, it's important to remember that exercise at such a time is an excel-lent activity. The very act of sweating is an effective antidote to menstrual bloating, which is a form of water retention.

FACT

Menstruation need not interfere with your competitive urges. Many women runners report little to no change in racing results when they run competitively during their menstrual period. Even when they run with mental and/or physical discomfort, running seems to make women feel better in the end.

Many women runners who exercise regularly find they suffer less-severe cramps and are less affected by menstrual side effects than are women who do not exercise. The other side is that there are women who no lon-ger menstruate regularly or at all because they overdo exercise relative to their caloric intake in both training and racing. Even though this might not seem like such a bad thing, infrequent or irregular menstrual cycles, called *amenorrhea,* can lead to an early onset of osteoporosis and interfere with childbearing. It is strongly recommended that women runners discuss their running habits and their monthly menstrual cycle with their doctor from time to time to make sure they are neither overdoing exercise nor neglecting important health concerns.

Osteoporosis and Menopause

Osteoporosis, a disease of brittle bones that affects a great many women, can mean the unfortunate end to a running career. The jarring action of running or a quick fall can cause a fracture. When bone mass begins to decline around the age of 35, women become vulnerable to osteoporosis. If undetected, the process can accelerate after menopause. However, young women with diets low in iron and calcium who place too much stress on their bodies can also contract this disease.

Osteoporosis cannot be reversed. If an affected woman detects osteoporosis early enough, she can slow the disease's progress with the help of her doctor. A calcium-rich diet is a primary way of retarding osteoporosis, as are weight-bearing exercises such as walking and running. The appropriate amount of stress increases bone density, thereby strengthening bones. If you are a woman runner, you should discuss osteoporosis with your doctor at your next medical appointment.

Menopause

Menopause is a difficult time for some women, less so for others. Although it can involve deep mood swings, hot flashes, and other discomforts, it need not discourage women from running. There has been no conclusive evidence that running (or other kinds of exercise) increases or decreases the main effects of menopause. However, there is little doubt that exercise is a wonderful antidote to stress, depression, anxiety, and a host of other less desirable emotions.

Since menopause can take as long as ten years to complete its cycle, many aging women lose their desire and motivation to continue running. Regardless, countless dedicated women have continued running right through their entire menopause, never losing the enjoyment and richness that running brings to their lives. Again, consulting with your physician is your best way to run through menopause with the least amount of physical or mental discomfort.

Safety Tips for Women Runners

Though people like to think they live in an enlightened time when women are safe running by themselves, it's always a good idea to be aware of potentially unpleasant or dangerous situations. Here are common-sense suggestions to keep you safe. These tips also apply to men.

- Don't run in isolated areas, particularly after dark.
- Whenever possible, run with other people after dark.
- Vary your running routine. Don't run in the same place at the same time on the same days.
- Mix up your schedule so strangers can't anticipate when and where you run.
- Tell a family member, roommate, or friend of your route and approximately what time you expect to return.
- Bring a whistle, panic button device, or some other way to attract attention should a threat materialize.
- If possible, learn some self-defense tactics.

CHAPTER 20

On the Road All Year

Running is an activity you can do any time of the year. But running intelligently during different seasons requires forethought and specific strategies, especially during the extreme seasons of winter and summer. This chapter gives you the practical and health information necessary to deal with the elements and to enjoy running all year-round. If you use common sense, dress correctly, stay hydrated, and follow the normal protocol of letting someone know your running route and not overexerting yourself on your training runs, you should be able to stick to a training schedule through all seasons.

Running in Cold Weather

Depending on your geographic location, winter may not be an optimal time to plan a dramatic increase in mileage or to add speed work to your training regimen. Cold and icy conditions make running more hazardous. Slipping, muscle guarding (a muscle spasm in response to a painful stimulus), and cool muscles can contribute to hamstring and groin pulls.

Cold Weather Strategies

Warm up well before going out, and be especially careful when running on surfaces that are wet or icy. Shorten your stride, and run slower than usual. When running just after a winter storm, if you have a choice of running on ice or snow, choose the snow. You will be less likely to slip because the traction is better.

To help yourself keep warm, a good strategy to remember is to run out against the wind and return with the wind at your back. The greater the amount of cold air passing over your exposed body surface, the faster your body will cool off. By running against the wind, you'll be facing the most environmental stress when you are fresh, maybe running faster, and you will not be soaked with perspiration during the first half of the run. You will tend to stay warmer on the return leg when running with the wind to your back, especially if you have been sweating. The wind behind you will also help keep you moving.

Dressing for Cold Weather Runs

It is important to protect all areas of your body from exposure. This includes your face, head, hands, feet, legs, arms, and chest. Also, don't forget your other more delicate parts: Men should consider investing in underwear with an insulated front panel for extra protection.

To protect your feet, which conduct cold through the soles of your running shoes as they strike the cold trails or roads, wear dry socks made of a wicking material. Acrylic material can wick moisture away, which prevents moisture from forming around your feet while you run and turning to ice when you stop running. You can cover a thin inner sock with a thicker outer sock, provided this doesn't pad your foot so much that you can barely squeeze your foot into your shoe. Immediately following your run, change into a dry pair of socks.

Nike Dri-FIT®, Capilene®, Varitherm®, Cocona®, and Coolmax® are names of fabrics designed to keep your body either warm and dry or cool and dry. No longer is it necessary to wear multiple layers of T-shirts, sweatshirts, or even a parka to stay warm in the coldest weather. Although you still need to layer, today's materials are less bulky, more comfortable, and better designed to protect against the elements. Cotton fabric will hold moisture and lose its insulating properties. Wool and today's Smartwool® will continue to insulate and keep you warm even when they are wet.

A combination to keep you toasty and dry consists of a thin layer of synthetic material to pull moisture away from your body, covered with fleece for insulation, then topped with a breathable, waterproof layer.

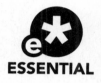

ESSENTIAL

Your skin is the part of your body most exposed to environmental conditions. Nourish and protect it by staying hydrated (whether it's hot or cold out) and wear sunscreen when you run. Sunblock and moisturizer help prevent a weathered face.

A facemask or scarf further minimize exposure, especially of the thin skin on your face, and a hat and gloves are musts. For your head, choose a lightweight synthetic fabric that wicks away moisture and won't itch. A fleece or Smartwool® gator will keep your neck warm, which can make all the difference when running in cold weather. For hands in relatively mild temperatures, some runners wear painters gloves as recommended by Bill Rogers. For colder weather, you can wear inner polypropylene gloves with an outer layer of mittens. Choose a soft and absorbent material that can also go in the wash, since cold air hitting the warmer air from your nose will cause your nose to run, in which case wiping it with the back of your hand is the most practical solution.

For your legs, you can add sweatpants over polypropylene tights, or if it is exceptionally cold wear Gore-Tex® or nylon pants on the outer layer.

Running in Hot Weather

The best defense against heat is hydration. Therefore, when the temperature goes up, so should your fluid intake. Water should always be your number one drink of choice. Drink before, during, and after you run. Drink before you go to sleep, and drink when you wake up. In short, drink water often throughout the day, regardless of weather conditions. In general, you should drink at least eight glasses of water a day. When it's really hot out, you can easily double this amount. However, be mindful not to drink excessive amounts of water; avoid hyponatremia.

Always drink before you run and try to drink about 8 ounces every 25–30 minutes while you run. Although just water is fine for runs of up to an hour, you will find that sports drinks maintain your performance level for runs over 1 hour. Most popular sport drinks have a low level of electrolytes and also contain carbohydrates (both simple and more complex polymers) to help speed up glycogen replacement.

Please don't count coffee, beer, or other caffeinated and alcoholic beverages as part of your daily tally of fluids. Although research has shown that caffeine does seem to enhance performance, depending on how long your run is, remember that a caffeine buzz can turn into a wilt. You may not want to skip coffee before you run, but just make sure you drink plenty of water, too.

Immediately following exercise, muscles are most receptive to absorbing carbohydrates (which later convert to the stored energy glycogen), which is why you'll often find bagels and fruit offered at the end of a race. But don't forget to meet your overall fluid replacement needs with water as well as with fluids containing ample carbohydrates, such as fruit or vegetable juices.

To help you stay hydrated during long, hot summers of running, consider stopping at every water fountain you pass and taking a drink. Don't forget to give yourself a minimum of two weeks to fully acclimate to the heat. The best way to do this is by running a slow 3–4 miles, making sure you have enough water. Gradually increase your distance and cumulative time running.

Also try combining indoor treadmill running with outside running to get more distance on really hot days. During the first hot, humid days of spring and summer, slowly build your mileage to acclimate to these conditions before considering running at a faster pace. In fact, many seasoned runners put their fast-paced efforts on hold until cooler weather returns. Additionally, try to miss the heat by running early in the morning or late at night. Remember, though, that if you run early in the morning, you may experience more humidity. And, of course, consider using an indoor treadmill on the worst days. That way you can get a workout with a few more miles in a cooler environment.

FACT

Perspiration and evaporation of perspiration are the primary means for the body to cool during exercise. Sweat glands become active as body-core temperature rises. One liter of sweat is generated during the expenditure of about 500 kilocalories (kcal). Skin blood flow also increases significantly during exercise. Blood flowing near the surface enhances cooling by both conduction and convection.

Heat-Induced Illness

Several illnesses can be induced by heat. The first, heat exhaustion, is caused by dehydration. The symptoms include chills, lightheadedness, dizziness, headache, and nausea. Body temperature usually rises to between 100–102 degrees Fahrenheit, and profuse sweating is evident. To treat heat exhaustion, move to a cool, shaded area, call an ambulance, and drink fluids until help arrives.

ALERT

Make sure you are aware of any medical conditions you have or of any medications you are taking that affect your tolerance for exercise in the heat. Medical conditions affecting heat tolerance include diabetes, high blood pressure, anorexia nervosa, bulimia, obesity, and fever.

Heat stroke, a serious heat-induced illness, is caused by a sudden failure of the body's thermoregulatory system. Not only is this dangerous, but it can also be fatal. Heat stroke initially presents like heat exhaustion but can rapidly progress to more serious neurological symptoms, such as disorientation, loss of consciousness, and seizures. Body temperature can rise higher than 104 degrees Fahrenheit. Sweating is often absent, but the skin can be quite moist from earlier perspiration. The pulse of a person afflicted with heat stroke is usually more than 160 beats per minute, and blood pressure may be low.

If you are suffering from heat stroke, your core temperature must be reduced immediately. Kidney damage (acute nephropathy) occurs in about 35 percent of cases. This is a result of *rhabdomyolysis* (muscle breakdown) and *myoglobinuria* (excretion of muscle breakdown products in the urine), which contribute to kidney injury. Liver damage is also evident when liver enzymes are measured following heat stroke. Oftentimes getting packed in ice reduces core temperature. Heat stroke is a medical emergency. It is vital that you seek immediate medical attention.

Avoiding Heat Stress Injury

To avoid heat exhaustion or heat stroke, drink plenty of fluids (preferably water) 25–30 minutes before exercise and then 8 ounces every 25–30 minutes while exercising. After exercising, drink more fluids than you think you need, especially if you are over the age of 40. Don't wait until you feel thirsty; by that time you're already dehydrated. Drinking fluids while you exercise as well as when you're finished helps speed your recovery.

You can also protect yourself from the heat by gradually building up your tolerance for running in warmer weather. Stay fit, and don't overestimate your level of fitness. Individuals with a higher VO_2 max (the amount of oxygen delivered to your muscles every minute) are more tolerant of heat than those with a lower VO_2 max.

ALERT

If you run when it's dark (at any time of the year), wear a reflective garment. Reflective garments are made of high-tech materials that provide safety, comfort, and temperature control to keep you cool in the summer and warm in the winter.

Dressing Cool for the Heat

Even if you feel like you don't want to wear anything at all when it's really hot out, don't make that mistake! The worst thing to do is to overheat your body and then, with no protection, expose it to rapid cooling. This can cause lightheadedness and dizziness or a more serious heat injury.

When running in the heat, wear lightweight fabrics that wick away moisture, support your body, and neutralize odor. There are all sorts of comfortable and fashionable shorts and tops available for men and women. Workout apparel these days is about comfort, fit, performance, and style.

As for upper body wear, women can opt for a colorful sports bra and men a breezy fabric singlet. Thin, absorbent socks can keep your feet from getting too sweaty and minimize blisters. To keep sweat from dripping into your eyes, you might want to wear a headband or a visor. Even though baseball caps shield the sun, they trap heat—something to consider on hot, humid days. Don't forget to apply heavy-duty sunscreen, especially on your face.

ESSENTIAL

It is important to remember that environmental comfort is a highly individualized matter. By experimenting with a variety of layering apparel, you can learn how to dress effectively and comfortably for facing the elements. This in turn will enable you to train both safely and consistently.

Running Indoors

Running outside in inclement weather prepares you for races, which don't stop for the weather (save, of course, for extreme weather like thunderstorms, hurricanes, and snowstorms). Running outside regardless of the weather is a healthy and invigorating experience.

Even so, running indoors is reliable, convenient, limits your exposure to outside risks, and can be more sociable if you choose it to be. If there's a school or college nearby that has an indoor track you can use, consider doing so. It's a nice alternative to running on a treadmill at home or at the gym. Be careful, though, as some indoor tracks are shorter than ⅛ of a mile. Short tracks have more turns, which can adversely affect your knees, ankles, and hips. Look for tracks that are longer than at least ⅛ mile, and check whether it's permissible to change directions halfway through your run, which is better for your legs. Some tracks prefer that everyone run in the same direction.

A treadmill is a good option for indoor running and can be done at home or at a gym or club. There are new indoor treadmills coming to market all the time. The best indoor treadmill is the one that works for you. Experiment with several before you hone in on one, and be receptive to trying new ones that show up in your gym.

QUESTION

How do I determine my miles per hour?
Pace is the number of minutes it takes to travel 1 mile. To determine your pace, divide 60 by your treadmill speed in miles per hour. For example: If your treadmill speed equals 3.5 mph, divide 60 by 3.5. You are covering a mile in 17 minutes.

Running on treadmills is recommended when you have no choice and you don't want to miss a workout. The treadmill's convenience is wonderful, but ultimately it is not the best method to train for long-distance running. Those in training for a marathon still need to do a large percentage of running on roads, particularly with those all-important long runs. As you run indoors, remember to focus on your form. When you exercise, proper posture and technique are essential to maximizing your effort and avoiding injury. Many runners respect the importance of posture and mechanics when doing outside sports but give little thought to these when exercising indoors on equipment.

Using the Treadmill

Most commercial equipment in health clubs is clearly labeled with instructions. But if you are still unclear about how to use the equipment, ask the staff for assistance. If you are going to buy a piece of equipment, make sure you get a demonstration on how to properly use and maintain it (along with a warranty and instruction manual if buying from a retail store).

Here are some tips for using a treadmill:

- Learn how to use it *before* you use it.
- Use manual mode for complete control of the intensity (speed, elevation, and resistances).
- Pay attention to your intensity level and your use of distractions to pass the time (music, reading, talking, thinking) so you don't overdo it.
- Drink fluids during exercise to stay hydrated.
- Use a fan to keep from getting overheated.

Once you get used to the feeling of the ground moving beneath your feet, you will truly appreciate running on a treadmill. The treadmill is obedient and will keep the speed and elevation steady at the levels you set. The speed and elevation settings determine the treadmill's intensity. You can either control the settings yourself through manual mode or experiment with pre-programmed workouts. Many home models allow you to program your own workouts and keep them in memory as a preprogrammed workout.

Learn how to control your treadmill:

- Know where the stop button is located.
- Practice grabbing the handrail and standing on the nonmoving side panels before stopping the machine.
- Stay focused and avoid turning your body or looking directly down at your feet.
- Keep children and pets away from the treadmill and from the operating key.
- Position the back of the treadmill away from a wall so that you do not bump into it.

Shopping for a Treadmill

Commercial treadmills can accommodate persons of most body weights; home models are typically built to withstand body weights not greater than 250 pounds. If you presently walk and are planning to eventually run on the treadmill, a minimum horsepower of 1.5–2.0 is recommended. Be sure to ask the salesperson whether the machine has incline capability. Being able to vary the incline gives you more variety in the type of workouts you can do (or progress to doing).

Noise is difficult to detect on a showroom floor, but listen for it anyway. Compare the store surroundings with those where you will put your machine. If it seems a bit noisy in the showroom and you plan to put the treadmill in a small room with little insulation, expect that it will be even louder at home.

Take measurements to make sure you have enough room for the treadmill you are considering, and for safety purposes, avoid positioning the treadmill with its back close to a wall. One small misstep and you could be thrown with an unplanned back injury—as well as finding yourself in need of some home remodeling.

Safety Features

You absolutely want an emergency pull/stop mechanism ("kill switch," which stops the machine). In the event that you unexpectedly fall (or move more than a few feet from the front handle of the treadmill), a light emergency cord connected to the treadmill control panel would disengage and instantly stop the motor. Some people prefer to wear this chord clipped onto their clothing; others prefer that it rest within reach on top of the treadmill. Either way, this mechanism is an effective and valuable safety feature.

ESSENTIAL

Do not waste your money on nonelectrical or human-powered treadmills. The movement of the belt is stiff, sluggish, and uneven, which doesn't feel like something you'd want to stay on for more than a minute. The mental and physical energy spent on this kind of treadmill is better spent on one more enjoyable and easier to use.

Another safety feature preferred by many people is a treadmill railing. Front rails are best; side rails are steadying but for some can get in the way during exercise. If you aren't sure which you prefer, this is another reason to check out several treadmills and feel the differences between models.

Deck, Speed, and Other Features

Deck flexibility makes a difference in how your bones and joints feel in response to the treadmill's impact. There is no standard word to describe how flexible the deck is, but you need to inquire whether the treadmill you are considering has such a system. Good treadmills have some type of flexible deck system.

You also want a smooth belt action, which means that the machine can pull its own weight (and yours) without hesitation or knocking. Ask what the maximum speed and maximum elevation of the machine are. If you consistently run a blazing 6-minute mile or faster, some treadmills cannot match your speed, and therefore you would not want to buy them.

The control panel displays such measurements as your distance, speed, calories burned, elevation, and heart rate, as well as your programmable workouts. The more components you want to see displayed on the console, the higher the price. But do not let that discourage you. Envision yourself walking and running on the treadmill for years to come and think about how much enjoyment and motivation you will derive from knowing how you perform in those seemingly trivial areas that the console displays.

Finally, note which creature comforts (if any) are important to you, such as cup and magazine holders. Make a list of questions and bring it with you when shopping so all your concerns are addressed before buying.

But It's a Vacation!

True, vacations are times when you leave the stresses and worries of your daily routine behind and indulge in the good life. For many people that means rest, relaxation, and fun like sightseeing, dining out, dancing, sunbathing, and other leisure activities. Do you see running on this list? No. Would most of your friends call you crazy if you told them you were looking forward to running your 5 miles a day on your trip to the Grand Canyon? Probably, but remember: It's your time off, not theirs!

Reasons to Run on Vacation

Think of it this way. If you have set up a running routine to get in shape and lose weight, you're probably already seeing results and enjoying running by now. When you go on vacation and indulge in big meals, drinking, and extra sleep, those pounds and inches will come back in no time—unless, of course, you can get in a few runs. Even short runs will keep your metabolism humming and ensure that you don't regress. You'll enjoy that piña colada even more knowing you've earned it through aerobic exercise.

If you're in training for a half-marathon or marathon, not getting miles in for a couple of weeks could throw you off. You don't want to undermine all the hard work and training miles you've put in by not keeping up with your running during a trip.

"I Was Going to Run, But . . ."

Many runners have given any number of reasons for not performing their workouts when out of town. Although it's great to have fun and break away from your normal routine when traveling, it's important not to let your running go on vacation, particularly if you're training for an event just a few short weeks away. Feelings of worry and guilt can arise upon viewing those blank spaces in your training log. If only you had done things differently!

Planning ahead greatly increases the likelihood that you will maintain your training while away. Long before your departure, your first step is to research all your options concerning when and where you can run.

Oftentimes, running first thing in the morning proves the best solution, particularly when your agenda is quite full. But it's also important to be realistic. If you expect to be partying well past midnight at a wedding reception, will you have the self-discipline and motivation to follow through with your plan to run early the next morning?

If you're traveling with family members, it's important to consider their needs. Are there activities they can do while you're out running? Who will be watching the kids for the hour or so that you're away? How will you work it out so that your partner also has some private time?

Lodging Considerations

Where you decide to stay can also affect the likelihood you will run when out of town. Hotels that have fitness centers equipped with treadmills make running easy. Some accommodating hotels in big cities have mapped out running routes of various distances that begin and end at their front door. If your hotel doesn't have workout facilities on-site, ask management whether they have special arrangements with a nearby gym that their guests can use at reduced rates or even for free.

If you prefer staying at an economy motel when away, select one located adjacent to residential neighborhoods or on a road with sidewalks and light traffic so that it will be both safe and convenient to run directly from your room. You can always hop in your car to run in another part of town if you don't feel comfortable with your motel's location.

If you will be staying at the home of friends or relatives, let them know in advance that you plan to run so they will be supportive of your training. They might be able to suggest a good running route nearby or have runner friends who would welcome you to join them.

ALERT

If there is absolutely no way to fit in a workout during your weekend getaway, modify your training schedule to fit in those important runs before leaving. Be sure not to cluster too many days of running back-to-back, though, since doing so can lead to injury.

If you're going away to rekindle the romance in your relationship and your significant other is not a runner, remind him or her (and yourself) that regular exercise helps you feel and look better. It improves your circulation, overall health, energy level, mental acuity, and appetite—all important for a healthy sex life! In fact, perhaps the two of you can begin participating in exercise together while away. It's an ideal way to bond and have fun.

Run to See the Sights

Besides the very important and real benefits of maintaining your fitness regimen while you're on the road, the greatest satisfaction in running away from home is in exploring new places, runners often proclaim. Let's face it, there's nothing like running through a new neighborhood to reinvigorate your runs. It's fun to see how people in other parts of the country (and the world) decorate their homes and yards, configure their streets, and go about their daily lives. Not only are you getting your exercise in, but you're getting an up-close-and-personal look at a new part of the world. You'll be amazed at how invigorating this is.

Don't be surprised if you start remembering your trips by the runs you took instead of the meals you ate, the museums you visited, even the family stories you heard for the first time. When you're on your run, the time is yours. Even if only a quick 20 minutes, running on your own in a new place revives all your senses.

ESSENTIAL

If you've gotten into the good habit of keeping a running log or journal, this will come in handy when you're traveling. Take notes about what you have liked best about your run and what you have liked least. In this way, your running log becomes your travel journal.

Planning for Safety

If adventure is one side of the equation in running while away from home, safety is the other. Because as exciting as it is to be in new places, the truth is that you're not on familiar territory. Taking a wrong turn on foot somewhere can get you lost more easily than you think. If you don't speak the native language, have no map with you, or find yourself in the dark, you could be in big trouble. And though most runners agree that it's particularly gratifying to do some of these runs alone, running by yourself exposes you to more dangers—anything from twisting your ankle while running on a trail to accidentally running into the bad part of town.

Use Common Sense

Such frightening scenarios are easily avoided by following common sense safety rules. First, trust your instincts. If a business trip on a limited budget puts you in a hotel where there's nothing but strip malls and highways everywhere you look, you may have to either use the hotel gym or limit your run to laps around the parking lot. You certainly don't want to be running anywhere near a busy street or highway where cars are making quick turns or going at high speeds, not to mention feeling vulnerable in a setting like this.

Likewise, if you're a bit behind schedule and you get to your hotel, campsite, or bed and breakfast at dusk instead of earlier in the afternoon, however beautiful the setting, you should consider postponing your run until morning when you have the full advantage of daylight. Once you know a trail or an area and have gauged how far it is to run, then you may want to consider running at dusk. But *don't run anywhere new in the dark.*

FACT

There are certain areas in life where risk-taking can pay off big time. Running on the road is not one of them. If you wouldn't want a member of your family or one of your best friends to go out on the run you're considering, then don't do it yourself.

Another common sense safety rule is to leave a message with someone that you're going for a run. If you're traveling by yourself, you should leave a note in your hotel room, tent, or wherever you're staying. Indicate the time you are leaving and how long you expect to be out.

Another easy and practical thing to do is ask at the front desk whether there's a running trail accessible from the hotel. The staff is usually happy to tell you all about it, including whether there are loops of different lengths in case you want to do 3 miles one day and 10 another, for example. After getting the lowdown from the staff, you can let them know that you're going out on that trail and you expect the run to take you, say, a half-hour. Leave your name and your room number with the hotel personnel.

If you're traveling with others, make sure they know to expect you back within a certain time. Be generous with your estimate of the time but not overly so. You don't want them calling the police if you're not back in 45 minutes like you said because you decided to run a bit farther. On the other hand, you don't want them to figure you're just out enjoying yourself if you're not back within a few hours.

While on your run, carry identification with you. Write your name, home address, and phone number and the name, address, and phone number of the place where you're staying on a piece of paper that you can tuck into a pocket or gear holder. Don't wear anything that could make you a target, such as sparkling jewelry or your most expensive wristwatch.

You *must* wear or carry a timepiece with you. Best, of course, is your waterproof, lightweight sports watch that you've bought along with your other necessary gear for running. But if you have forgotten it, wear or carry your regular watch. Since you'll be setting off into the unknown, time is your best bearing. You might also carry your cell phone with you; not only can you tell time this way, but you can also call for help or directions if necessary.

ALERT

When running in a new place, you need a fanny pack or a wrist or ankle attachment that can hold a few small things like your hotel key, a few dollars in pocket change, and certainly identification. You'll need to feel comfortable but not conspicuous.

Plan to run 15–20 minutes out, then 15–20 minutes back. Because your senses are working overtime to take in everything new, running toward your destination will seem to take longer than your return trip. Keep an eye on the time. You'll feel like you've been running for longer than your watch or cell phone says, but when you get to the halfway point and start to head back, you'll enjoy reliving sights from the run out, and time will go by more quickly.

More Safety Tips

There's an excellent website called "Run the Planet" (*www.runtheplanet .com*) that's loaded with advice on where and when to run throughout the world. Here are some especially good tips from a section called "Stay Safe While Running" by the Hudson Mohawk Road Runners Club:

- Take a whistle with you.
- Know where police are usually to be found and where businesses, stores, and offices are likely to be open and active.
- Do not wear a radio/headset/earphones or anything that distracts you so that you are completely unaware of your environment.
- Take notice of who is ahead of you and who is behind you. Know where the nearest public sites are with some general activity—there is usually safety in numbers.

- When in doubt, follow your intuition and avoid potential trouble. If something seems suspicious, do not panic but run in a different direction.
- If the same car cruises past you more than once, take down even a partial license number and make it obvious that you are aware of its presence (but keep your distance).
- Do not approach a car to give directions or the time of day. Point toward the nearest police or information source, shrug your shoulders, but keep moving. If you feel you must respond, do it while moving.
- Do not panic. Do not run toward a more isolated area.
- Use discretion in acknowledging strangers. Be friendly, but keep your distance and keep moving.

Racing on the Road

One way to get an invigorating workout while on a business or pleasure trip is to enter a local race. Go online a few weeks before you're scheduled to leave and do a search for local running clubs in the area you're planning to visit. Go to their websites, and see what's on the race calendar. Call the contact person for the race to get more information on the size of the event, whether it's a hilly or flat course, whether there's a post-race party or expo, and so on. If you decide to do the race, ask for directions from the place where you'll be staying and ask how long it should take to get there.

FACT

Many cities have special races to celebrate holidays like Thanksgiving, Halloween, Memorial Day, Labor Day, and New Year's Day. New York City's Midnight Run on New Year's Eve draws thousands of runners from all over the world to run a 5K through Central Park at midnight, accompanied by fireworks and nonalcoholic champagne. It's an extremely festive and fun way to start a new year.

Marathoning Around the World

Why not do a really big race in a new place? That's what legions of marathoners from around the world choose to do. The many advantages are that you can get a good rate to travel and stay someplace for a week, you're traveling with like-minded folks, you don't have to worry too much about how much you eat while you're there (though, of course, you want to avoid foods that are too exotic, especially before the race), and you'll have an instant sightseeing tour.

It's easy to find information on running marathons in all corners of the world. Start at *www.runnersworld.com*, or buy *Runner's World* magazine, and you'll be on your way.

Finding a Running Club, at Home or Abroad

A Couple of Clicks Away

There are a number of excellent running clubs around the world that are easy to find, inexpensive to join, and that sponsor activities you can participate in on either a particular weekend or all year. Belonging to a running club is a good way to stay motivated, learn from others, meet people with similar interests, and participate in challenging events. Some clubs are big—like those associated with well-known marathons such as the Boston Athletic Club and the New York Road Runners Club. Sparsely populated areas have smaller clubs. Different clubs have different personalities.

Search via Goggle or Bing for "running club + [the name of your town, state initials]" (for example, "running club + Kimberton, PA"). You're bound to find a lot of interesting sites even if they aren't what you were originally looking for.

Clubs in the United States

In the United States, the best place to start is with the granddaddy of them all, the Road Runners Club of America (RRCA) at *www.rrca.org*. Not only can you find local and national club listings through the RRCA, you can get an idea of what's happening with running across the country. To find clubs in the state where you live or a state you're planning to visit, you can go straight to a map on their website, click on the state, and immediately access a list of all the running clubs in that state. The RRCA's contact information is:

Road Runners Club of America (National Office)
1501 Lee Highway, Suite 140
Arlington, VA 22209
Phone: (703) 525-3890
www.rrca.org

Clubs in Canada

Like the United Sates, Canada has lots of running clubs that offer organized events for their members and guests. One of the top sites to search for clubs in Canada and in other countries (as well as in the United States) is the "Running Network" at:

Running Network, LLC
www.runningnetwork.com

Outside the United States and Canada

"Run the Planet" at *www.runtheplanet.com* provides an excellent international directory. If you search on the site for running clubs, you'll be directed to pages of national and international listings. Besides the United States and Canada, you can look up clubs in Africa, Antarctica, Asia, Europe, Oceania, and South America. In the "Race Calendar" section, you'll find information on races in Austria, Belgium, Switzerland, Serbia and Montenegro, the Czech Republic, Germany, Denmark, Spain, Finland, France, the United Kingdom, Greenland, Greece, Hungary, Ireland, Iceland, Italy, Luxembourg, Latvia, the Netherlands, Norway, Poland, Portugal, Romania, Russia, Sweden, and Slovenia. What's to stop you? "Run the Planet" is also a treasure trove of information about all aspects of running, including its history.

APPENDIX B

Magazines and Books on Running

Magazines

With the explosion of information available on the Internet, you'd think magazines and books would be obsolete. However, the ever-expanding selection of magazines, periodicals, and books is a testament to the fact that nothing quite beats the tactile experience of hands-on reading.

Sure you can find all kinds of information online, even race calendars, but there's nothing like finding it all in one place in a running magazine. Some of the most popular and well-known running magazines are listed below. Check 'em out!

Runner's World—**"The worldwide authority on running information"**
www.runnersworld.com

Running Journal—**"The source for road racing and fitness news in the Southeast"**
www.running.net

Running Research News—**"A monthly newsletter which keeps sports-active people up-to-date on the latest information about training, sports nutrition, and sports medicine."**
www.rrnews.com

Running Times—**"The runner's best resource"**
www.runningtimes.com

Marathon & Beyond—**"Run longer, better, smarter"**
www.marathonandbeyond.com

National Masters News
www.nationalmastersnews.com

TrailRunner—**Helps runners of all ages and abilities experience the outdoors and achieve a healthier lifestyle through off-road running"**
www.trailrunnermag.com

Ultrarunning—**"The voice of the ultrarunner"**
www.ultrarunning.com

Track & Field News—**"The Bible of the Sport Since 1948"**
www.trackandfieldnews.com

Books

If you enjoy reading about running, you already have one of the best books out there—this one! But like all sports and hobbies, running has produced a deep and wide body of works. The running library includes books on training for particular events, health and injuries, the psychology of running, and the pure enjoyment of running. This list is not all-inclusive, but it includes classics by Dr. George Sheehan, Bob Glover, Jeff Galloway, and Amby Burfoot.

General Training and Inspiration

Abshire, Danny. *Natural Running: The Simple Path to Stronger, Healthier Running.* (Velo Press, 2010)

Barrios, Dagny Scott. *Runner's World Complete Book of Women's Running: The Best Advice to Get Started, Stay Motivated, Lose Weight, Run Injury-Free, Be Safe, and Train for Any Distance.* (Rodale, 2007)

Battista, Garth, ed. *The Runner's Literary Companion: Great Stories and Poems about Running.* (Penguin Books, 1994)

Battista, Garth. *How Running Changed My Life: True Stories of the Power of Running.* (Breakaway Books, 2002)

Bingham, John. *No Need for Speed: A Beginner's Guide to the Joy of Running.* (Rodale, 2002)

Bloom, Marc. *Run with the Champions: Training Programs and Secrets of America's 50 Greatest Runners.* (Rodale, 2001)

Burfoot, Amby. *The Principles of Running: Practical Lessons from My First 100,000 Miles.* (Rodale, 1999)

Burfoot, Amby. *The Runner's Guide to the Meaning of Life: What 35 Years of Running Has Taught Me about Winning, Losing, Happiness, Humility, and the Human Heart.* (Daybreak Books, 2000)

Burfoot, Amby. *Runner's World Complete Book of Running: Everything You Need to Run for Fun, Fitness, and Competition, Revised Ed.* (Rodale, 2009)

Burfoot, Amby. *Runner's World Complete Book of Beginning Running.* (Rodale, 2005)

Chase, Adam and Nancy Hobbs. *The Ultimate Guide to Trail Running, 2nd Edition.* (Globe Pequot Press, 2010)

Clark, Nancy. *Nancy Clark's Sports Nutrition Guidebook.* (Human Kinetics, 2008)

Couch, Jean. *The Runner's Yoga Book: A Balanced Approach to Fitness.* (Rodmell Press, 1990)

Craythorn, Dennis and Rich Hanna. *The Ultimate Runner's Journal: Your Daily Training Partner and Log.* (Marathon Publishing, 1998)

Daniels, Jack, PhD. *Daniels' Running Formula, 2nd Edition.* (Human Kinetics, 2005)

Dreyer, Danny. *ChiRunning: A Revolutionary Approach to Effortless, Injury-Free Running* (2nd edition). (Fireside, 2009)

Ellis, Joe and Joe Henderson. *Running Injury-Free: How to Prevent, Treat, and Recover from Dozens of Painful Problems.* (Rodale, 1994)

Fishpool, Sean. *Beginner's Guide to Long-Distance Running.* (Barrons, 2002)

Galloway, Jeff. *Galloway's Book on Running, 2nd Edition.* (Shelter Publications, 2002)

Galloway, Jeff. *Half-Marathon: You Can Do It, 4th Edition.* (Meyer & Meyer Sport, 2011)

Galloway, Jeff. *Jeff Galloway's Training Journal.* (Shelter Publications, 1998)

Galloway, Jeff and Barbara Galloway. *Women's Complete Guide to Running.* (Meyer & Meyer Sport, 2007)

Glover, Bob and Shelly-Lynn Florence Glover. *The Competitive Runner's Handbook: The Bestselling Guide to Running 5Ks Through Marathons.* (Penguin Books, 1999)

Glover, Bob. *The Runner's Handbook: The Best-Selling Classic Fitness Guide for Beginner and Intermediate Runners.* (Penguin Books, 1996)

Glover, Bob and Shelly-Lynn Florence Glover. *The Runner's Training Diary: For Fitness Runners and Competitive Racers.* (Penguin USA, 1997)

Henderson, Joe. *Best Runs: Lessons and Insights for Optimal Motivation, Training, and Racing.* (Human Kinetics, 1998)

Henderson, Joe. *Better Runs: 25 Years' Worth of Lessons for Running Faster and Farther.* (Human Kinetics, 1996)

Henderson, Joe. *Running 101: Essentials for Success.* (Human Kinetics, 2000)

Higdon, Hal. *Hal Higdon's How to Train: The Best Programs, Workouts, and Schedules for Runners of All Ages.* (Rodale, 1997)

Higdon, Hal. *Hal Higdon's Smart Running: Expert Advice on Training, Motivation, Injury Prevention, Nutrition, and Good Health.* (Rodale, 1998)

Higdon, Hal. *Run Fast: How to Beat Your Best Time Every Time.* (Rodale, 2000)

Higdon, Hal. *Run Fast: How to Train for a 5K or 10K Race.* (Rodale, 1992)

Kowalchik, Claire. *The Complete Book of Running for Women: Everything You Need to Know about Training, Nutrition, Injury Prevention, Motivation, Racing, and Much, Much More.* (Pocket Books, 1999)

Lundgren, Chris. *Runner's World Guide to Running and Pregnancy: How to Stay Fit, Keep Safe, and Have a Healthy Baby.* (Rodale, 2003)

Lynch, Jerry and Warren Scott. *Running Within: A Guide to Mastering the Body-Mind-Spirit Connection for Ultimate Training and Racing.* (Human Kinetics, 1999)

MacNeil, Ian. *The Beginning Runner's Handbook: The Proven 13-Week Walk/Run Program, Revised and Updated.* (Greystone Books, 2005)

Martin, David E., PhD, and Peter N. Coe. *Better Training for Distance Runners, 2nd Edition.* (Human Kinetics, 1997)

McDougall, Christopher. *Born to Run: A Hidden Tribe, Superatheletes, and the Greatest Race the World Has Ever Seen.* First Edition. (Alfred A. Knoph, 2009)

McMillan, Greg and Juliana Risner. *Zap! You're a Runner: The Beginning Runner's Guide to Fun and Fitness.* (Road Runner Sports, 1999)

Nelson, Kevin. *The Runner's Book of Daily Inspiration: A Year of Motivation, Revelation, and Instruction.* (McGraw-Hill, 1999)

Noakes, Tim, MD. *Lore of Running, 4th Edition.* (Human Kinetics/Oxford University Press, 2001)

Noakes, Tim and Stephen Granger. *Running Injuries: How to Prevent and Overcome Them.* (Oxford University Press, 2003)

Poulin, Kirsten, Christina Flaxel, MD, and Stan Swartz. *Trail Running: From Novice to Master.* (The Mountaineers Books, 2002)

Reese, Paul, with Joe Henderson. *The Old Man and the Road: Reflections While Completing a Crossing of All 50 States on Foot at Age 80.* (Keokee Company Publishing, 2000)

Runner's World Magazine. *Runner's World: Training Journal.* (Rodale, published annually)

Sheehan, George, MD. *Dr. George Sheehan on Getting Fit and Feeling Great: How to Feel Great 24 Hours a Day; Running and Being; This Running Life; Three Volumes in One.* (Wings Books, 1992)

Sheehan, George, MD. *George Sheehan on Running to Win: How to Achieve the Physical, Mental & Spiritual Victories of Running.* (Rodale, 1994)

Sheehan, George, MD. *Going the Distance: One Man's Journey to the End of His Life.* (Villard Books, 1996)

Sheehan, George, MD. *Personal Best: The Foremost Philosopher of Fitness Shares Techniques and Tactics for Success and Self-Liberation.* (Rodale, 1992)

Sheehan, George, MD. *Running and Being: The Total Experience.* (Second Wind II, 1998)

Svensson, Sharon L. *The Total Runner's Log: The Essential Training Tools for the Runner.* (Trimarket, 2001)

Will-Weber, Mark, ed. *The Quotable Runner: Great Moments of Wisdom, Inspiration, Wrongheartedness, and Humor, Revised.* (Breakaway Books, 2008)

Marathon Training

Bloch, Gordon Bakoulis. *How to Train for and Run Your Best Marathon.* (Fireside, 1993)

Galloway, Jeff. *Marathon: You Can Do It!* (Shelter Publications, 2001)

Griffin, Jane. *Nutrition for Marathon Running.* (Crowood Press, 2005)

Hanc, John. *The Essential Marathon: A Concise Guide to the Race of Your Life.* (Globe Pequot Press, 1996)

Henderson, Joe. *Marathon Training: A 100-Day Program to Your Best Race, 2nd Edition.* (Human Kinetics, 2003; updated for 2011 e-book)

Higdon, Hal. *Marathon: The Ultimate Training Guide, 4th Edition.* (Rodale, 2011)

Nerurkar, Richard. *Marathon Running: The Complete Training Guide.* (Globe Pequot, 2000)

Pfitzinger, Pete and Scott Douglas. *Advanced Marathoning, 2nd Edition.* (Human Kinetics, 2009)

Whitsett, David A., Forrest A. Dolgener, and Tanjala Mabon Kole. *The Non-Runner's Marathon Trainer.* (Master's Press, 1998)

Marathon History

Boeder, Robert B. *Beyond the Marathon: The Grand Slam of Trail Ultrarunning.* (Old Mountain Press, 1996)

Connelly, Michael. *26 Miles to Boston: The Boston Marathon Experience from Hopkinton to Copley Square.* (Globe Pequot Press, 2003)

Derderian, Tom. *The Boston Marathon: A Century of Blood, Sweat, and Cheers.* (Triumph Books, 2003)

Derderian, Tom. *Boston Marathon: The First Century of the World's Premium Running Event.* (Human Kinetics, 1994)

Lonergan, Tim. *Heartbreak Hill: The Boston Marathon Thriller.* Fiction. (Writers Club Press, 2002)

Martin, David E. and Roger W. H. Gynn. *The Olympic Marathon: The History and Drama of Sport's Most Challenging Event.* (Human Kinetics, 2000)

Rubin, Ron. *Anything for a T-shirt: Fred Lebow and the New York City Marathon, the World's Greatest Footrace.* (Syracuse University Press, 2004)

APPENDIX C

Running Online

Since the first edition of this book was released back in 2002, the Internet has exploded with new sites on running, from running barefoot to ultra-running. The sites included here are just a sampling of what's available online. If you search for something specific, like "running vacations," you're sure to tap into sites that seem custom-made for your interests.

A great place to begin your search is at *www.marathon training.com*. Go to the site map, and then look under "Running Links." There you will find a listing of useful sites that is continuously updated and added to. It includes general links, marathon training, online record-keeping, calendars, gear, and much more. The following annotated sites are some favorites as well.

General Sites

Cool Running—Race calendars, training tips, information on youth running; it's all here.
www.coolrunning.com

Runner's Web—A running and triathlon resource site.
www.runnersweb.com

Road Runners Club of America—Over 700 clubs and 180,000 members throughout America.
www.rrca.org

ChiRunning—The official source for all ChiRunning-related training, events, and advice.
www.chirunning.com

Barefoot Running—Harvard University's Skeletal Biology Lab.
www.barefootrunning.fas.harvard.edu

On the Run—Your online source for the long-distance running community.
www.ontherunevents.com

Running Network, LLC—The most comprehensive source of information for grassroots runners online.
www.runningnetwork.com

Runner's World Magazine—It's not just a website for the magazine; it's a world of advice for runners.
www.runnersworld.com

Dr. Stephen M. Pribut's Sports Medicine Page—A site with lots of helpful sports medicine information.
www.drpribut.com

Marathon Training Websites

State of the Art Marathon Training—Offers a wide range of running topics designed to meet the needs of the beginner to the advanced competitor.
www.marathontraining.com

Hal Higdon on the Run—Provides advice from a foremost marathon competitor and trainer.
www.halhigdon.com

Jeff Galloway's Marathon Training Program—Check out the official site from the guy who started a marathoning revolution.
www.jeffgalloway.com

USA FIT—"Change your life" with helpful marathon tips.
www.usafit.com

Association of International Marathons and Distance Races (AIMS)—Tap into the international running community here.
www.aims-association.org

Ultra-Running

Ultra-Running Resource Site—Gives you information on every aspect of ultra-running.
www.ultrunr.com

Official website of the Western States Endurance Run (100 Miles)—A great site to look at to understand what's involved in an ultra endurance run.
www.ws100.com

American Ultrarunning Association—A resource for news and information on ultra-running in the United States.
www.americanultra.org

Stan "Runs 100s" Jensen—An ultra-runner's personal website, full of useful links and information.
www.run100s.com

Ultrarunning Online—Provides interesting articles and photos for ultra-runners.
www.ultrarunning.com

Index

Accessories, 34–35, 215–16, 224–25, 237–38
Achilles tendonitis
    Achilles tendon rupture, 173–74
    biomechanics of, 160, 170–71
    causes of, 171–72
    shin splints and, 190
    shoes and, 160, 162
    treating, 172
Achilles tendon rupture, 173–74
    causes of, 173
    diagnosing, 173
    steroid injections and, 173
    treating, 173
Analgesic creams, 224–25
Ankle injuries. See Achilles tendonitis; Injuries (foot and ankle)
Anterior shin splints, 182–85
Arc Trainer®, 91
Arms and hands, 83
Athlete's foot (tinea pedis), 176–77
Attitude
    adjusting, for running, 3–4
    excuses for not running, 2–3

Barefoot running, 119–32
    about: overview of, 119
    adaptation time, 130. See also retraining for
    age considerations, 123
    ChiRunning® vs., 144–45
    debates about, 120

defined, 120
    energy return, 123
    hypomobility, hypermobility and, 124
    injuries and, 129–31
    Matthew Walsh progression, 127
    mechanics of, 125–26
    medical considerations, 124
    plantar fasciitis and, 121–22, 125
    popularity of, 120–21
    preparation exercises, 126
    retraining for, 124–28
    running lightly, 124–25
    running shoes and, 120–22, 123
    safety concerns, 123, 124
    sample progressions, 127–28
    shifting load, 125
    shoes designed for, 131–32
    Vibram USA recommendations, 128
Benefits of running, 5–10
    focusing on, 5
    physical, 7–8
    psychological, 8–9
    social, 9
    talking to other runners about, 5–6
Blisters
    fungal infections and, 176
    lubrication to avoid, 216
    shoe fit and, 29, 161, 196
    socks and, 32, 224, 265
Books and magazines, 278–81

Bras, 33, 265
Breathing, 75–76, 137
Burnout, avoiding, 88, 223, 246

Caffeine, 45, 197–98, 225, 262
Carbohydrates. See Nutrition
Cardiac output, 7
Cell phones, 62, 207, 237–38, 274
ChiRunning®, 133–45
    about: overview of, 133–45
    adjusting to, 142–44
    aligning yourself, 138
    Balance in Motion principle, 136
    barefoot running vs., 144–45
    best way to learn, 143–44
    Body Sensing skill, 137
    Breathing skill, 137
    characteristics and principles, 134–36
    Chi-Skills, 137–38
    elements of, 136–41
    feeling the Chi, 142
    Focusing Your Mind skill, 137
    Gradual Progress principle, 135–36
    lean and, 138–39
    mindfulness and, 141
    movement, 143
    "Needle in Cotton" principle, 135
    pelvic rotation and, 140–41
    physical therapy and, 144
    Relaxation skill, 138
    rhythm of, 139–40

ChiRunning®—continued
shifting gears, 140
striding and landing, 139
T'ai Chi and, 134, 135–36
using your Y'chi, 141
your "column" and, 138
Climbing walls, 92
Clothing, 18, 20, 32–33, 215–16, 224, 237, 260–61, 264–65
Clubs, running, 105, 277
Cold weather, 260–61
Commitment tools, 13–14. See also Success tips
Cool-down routine, 112
Cost of running, 3
Cramps, avoiding, 198, 225, 242
Cramps, menstrual, 255
Creams and lubricants, 216, 224–25, 237
Cross-training. See also Weight training
about: overview of, 87
climbing walls, 92
cycling, 89–90
exercise machines, 91–92
ideal activities, 89–92
meditation, meditative running and, 153–54
Pilates and, 148
pros, cons, and precautions, 88–89
Reiki and, 155–56
water activities, 90–91
yoga and, 148–53
Cycling, 89–90

Deep-water running, 91
Downhill running, 85–86
Dry heaves or vomiting, 184–85

Elliptical trainers, 91
Endorphins, 8–9, 170
Ergometers, 92

Excuses for not running, 2–3
Exercise machines, 91–92. See also Treadmills

Fartlek workouts, 106–7, 114, 115
Female athletes. See Women (and girls) and running
Fiber, 42
Fitness and health
benefits of running, 5–10
establishing foundation for, 19–22
focusing on, 5
striving for, 2
5K Races, 193–204
about: overview of, 193
after the race, 203
atmosphere of, 194
basics of, 194–95
eating and drinking for, 196–98
injury during, 202
pacing and staying relaxed, 201–2
physical preparation, 199
psychological issues and concerns, 199–200
during the race, 200–203
readying watch for, 201
running after 10K, 209
start of, 200–201
strategy and goal setting, 195
supplements during, 203
themed races, 203–4
water stops, 202
week before, 195–96
Food. See Nutrition
Footstrikes, 76–80. See also Pronation and underpronation (supination)
ChiRunning® and, 139
flat, heel, and toe, 79–80
foot type and, 78
heel-ball and ball-heel-toe, 80
mechanics of foot and, 77–78
toes' role in, 78–79
Form. See Mechanics of running

Gait. See also Mechanics of running
anatomy of, 166
stance and swing phases of, 166–67
Goals
announcing, 13
defining specifically, 14–15
for 5Ks, 195
for marathons, 229–32, 241, 243, 246
notebook for. See Notebook (journal)
race strategy and, 195
for 10Ks and half-marathons, 206, 207

Half-marathons. See also Long runs
about: overview of, 205
after the race, 216–17
cooling down after, 216
eating and drinking after, 216
eating and drinking for, 214–15
mileage buildup for, 209–10
shoes, apparel, accessories for, 215–16
stretching after, 217
training schedules, 210
Heat-induced illness, 263–64
Heel spurs, 177–78, 179
Hill repeats, 105–6
Hills, running up and down, 85–86
Hydration. See Water and hydration
Hyponatremia, 49, 61, 198, 262

Ice, applying, 174–75
Iliotibial band syndrome (ITBS), 185–86
Imagery. See Visualization
Indoor running, 265–66
Inflammation, treating, 158–59
Injuries
ankle. See Injuries (foot and ankle)

barefoot running and, 129–31
effects of running on body and, 16
general guidelines, 170
leg. *See* Injuries (leg and other areas)
preventing. *See* Injury prevention
during races, 202
RICE for, 23, 174–75
running surface slants/camber and, 60
trail precautions, 60, 61–62
Injuries (foot and ankle), 169–80. *See also* Achilles tendonitis
about: overview of, 169
ankle sprains, 174–75
anterior ankle pain, 176
athlete's foot (tinea pedis), 176–77
biomechanics of foot and leg problems, 164–66
heel spurs, 177–78, 179
Morton's neuroma pain, 179–80
plantar fasciitis, 121–22, 125, 160–61, 177, 178–79
RICE for, 174–75
starting to exercise, 175
Injuries (leg and other areas), 181–91
about: overview of, 181
anterior shin splints, 182–85
biomechanics of foot and leg problems, 164–66
dry heaves or vomiting, 184–85
iliotibial band syndrome (ITBS), 185–86
medial shin splints (MTSS), 186–88
runner's knee, 188–90
shin splints, 190. *See also* anterior shin splints; medial shin splints (MTSS)
side stitches, 190–91
Injury prevention, 157–68

about: overview of, 157
anatomy of gait and, 165
basics of, 158–59
biomechanics of foot and leg problems, 164–66
gait phases and, 165–67
general guidelines, 61–62, 158
preventative rehabilitation program, 23
selecting sports physician, 167–68
shoes and, 159–62
stretching for, 163–64. *See also* Stretching
this book and, 3
treating inflammation, 158–59
Interval workouts, 108–11
about: overview of, 108
leg fatigue and, 109
pyramids and ladders, 110–11
repeat intervals, 110
target time and distances, 109–10
theory behind, 109
Inward focus. *See* Meditation and meditative running; Self-talk; Visualization; Yoga
Iron-deficiency anemia, 55–56
ITBS (Iliotibial band syndrome), 185–86

Journal. *See* Notebook (journal); Runner's (training) log

Knee injuries. *See* Injuries (leg and other areas)
Knee lift, 82

Long runs. *See also* Half-marathons; *Marathon references*
about: overview of, 222
areas of experimentation, 224–26
building up to, 223–24
definition and purpose of, 210–11, 222–23

easier, safer approach to, 223–24
food and eating considerations, 225, 234
with group, 212
hydration, 212–13
pace and time, 211–12
psychological issues, 213–14
running form and upper-body considerations, 212
shoes and, 224
Lubrication, to reduce chafing/blisters, 216, 225, 237

Magazines and books, 278–81
Marathon experience, 235–51. *See also* Ultra-running
about: overview of, 235
accessories for, 237–38
after the race, 244–46
aid stations, 241–42
cell phone for, 237–38
combating burnout, 246
cooling down after, 244
final hours before marathon, 239–40
life after, 246–48
lining up, 240
next race after, 246–48
on-course mental tips, 243–44
pacing, 211–12, 241
packing for out-of-town marathon, 236–38
physical preparation, 236
post-marathon evaluation, 245
preparing for. *See* Marathon preparation
pre-race morning checklist, 240
during the race, 240–44
report card checklist, 245–46
socializing, 242–43
staying on your feet after, 244–45
stretching after race, 244
supplementing, 242

Marathon experience—*continued*
  travel considerations, 236–39, 276
  visualizing results, 241
Marathon preparation, 219–34. *See also* Long runs
  about: overview of, 219
  advanced training schedule, 228
  anticipation, anxiety and, 233
  beginner training schedule, 227
  choosing marathon to enter, 220–21
  food and eating considerations, 225, 234
  history of marathons and, 220
  mental strategies, 232–34
  mental training, 229–32
  setting goals, 229–32
  stretching and, 233. *See also* Stretching
  tapering, 233
  training schedules, 226–28
  training websites, 283
  week before marathon, 233–34
Mechanics of running, 73–86
  about: overview of, 73
  anatomy of gait and, 165
  arms and hands, 83
  barefoot running and, 121–22
  breathing, 75–76
  footstrikes, 76–80
  form mistakes, 74, 121–22
  gait phases and, 165–67
  on hills (up and down), 85–86
  long run form and, 212
  posture, 84–85
  stride, 81–82
  style and mechanics, 74–75
Meditation and meditative running, 153–55
Menopause, 256
Menstruation, 255
Mental strategies, 232–34. *See also* Self-talk; Visualization

Mileage
  advanced buildup, 71
  building base, 21–22, 68
  buildup for half-marathon, 209–10
  buildup for 10K, 206–7
  buildup schedule, 69–70
  increasing, considerations, 206–7
  reverse taper, 247
  shoes and, 20, 37–38, 160, 161
  tapering, 68–69, 114, 196, 206, 233
  10 percent rule, 69
Minimalist shoes, 131–32
Mistakes, common, 22–24, 70–71
Morton's neuroma pain, 179–80
Motivation, 21, 62–63, 103, 229, 232, 233, 242, 243, 246. *See also* Commitment tools
Music, 34–35

Neuroma pain, 179–80
Notebook (journal), 14, 15, 19, 20, 38, 229, 272. *See also* Runner's (training) log
Nutrition, 39–56. *See also* Water and hydration
  about: overview of, 39
  balanced diet, 40–44
  before, during, after run, 46–51
  caffeine and, 45, 197–98, 225, 262
  calories and, 41
  carbohydrates, 22, 42, 44, 46, 48, 49, 50, 51, 53, 197, 234, 247, 262
  eating for running and racing, 44–46
  fats, 22, 43
  female athlete considerations, 53–56
  fiber, 42
  for 5Ks, 196–98
  for half-marathons, 214–15, 216
  "hitting the wall" and, 46
  hot weather and, 262

  hydration and. *See* Water and hydration
  hypoglycemia and, 47
  iron-deficiency anemia and, 55–56
  for long runs, 214–15, 216, 225
  for marathons, 225, 234, 237
  mindset, 40
  mix of nutrients, 22
  MyPlate system, 40–41, 46
  popular diets (Paleolithic and raw food), 52–53
  proteins, 22, 43
  supplemental energy sources (gels, bars, etc.), 203, 226, 237, 242
  typical runner diets, 51–52
  vitamins and minerals, 44

Orthotics, 31, 124, 129–30, 132, 172, 179, 189
Osteoporosis, 54, 93, 124, 255, 256

Pacing
  5Ks, 201–2
  long runs/marathons, 211–12, 241
Pelvic rotation, 140–41
Personal trainers, 67
Physician, selecting, 167–68
Pilates, 148
Plantar fasciitis, 121–22, 125, 160–61, 177, 178–79
Posture, 84–85
Precautions, 60–62
Pronation and underpronation (supination)
  barefoot running and, 129–30
  determining your foot type, 78
  gait phases and, 166–67
  heal spurs, plantar fasciitis and, 178
  ITBS and, 185
  mechanics of foot and, 77–78

MTSS and, 187–88
neuroma pain and, 180
orthotics and, 31, 172, 179
runner's knee and, 189–90
shin splints and, 183
shoe structure and, 29, 129, 160–61
Proteins. *See* Nutrition
Psychological benefits of running, 8–9
Pyramids and ladders, 110–11

Racing
5Ks. *See* 5K races
long runs. *See* Half-marathons; Marathon experience; Marathon preparation; Ultra-running
speed work benefits for, 103–4. *See also* Speed work
10Ks. *See* 10K races
Reasons for running. *See* Running
Recovery
after 10Ks and half-marathons, 209
after 5Ks, 203
after marathons, 246–48
avoiding injuries and, 158
defined, 109
drinking fluids speeding, 264
jogs, 107, 108, 110, 111, 114, 115
shortening time of, 136
techniques, 23–24, 49–51
Reiki, 155–56
Resources
magazines and books, 278–81
online, 282–83
running clubs, 277
Reverse taper, 247
RICE (Rest, Ice, Compression, and Elevation), 23, 174–75
Rowing machines (ergometers), 92
Runner's (training) log, 20–21, 35–38, 272. *See also* Notebook (journal)

Runner's knee, 188–90
about, 188
causes of, 188–89
treating, 189–90
Running
benefits of, 5–10
building relationship with, 4
effects on body, 16
not, excuses for, 2–3
striving for fitness, 2
Running clubs, 105, 277

Safety. *See also Injuries references*
barefoot running concerns, 123, 124
cross-training precautions, 88–89
general precautions, 60–62
planning for, when traveling, 272–75
tips for women, 257
treadmill, 268
Self-talk, 14, 207, 213, 229, 232, 243
Shin splints, anterior
about, 182
anterior compartment syndrome and, 182–83
defining, 190
office medical care, 184
runners at risk for, 183
self-care, 184
Shin splints, medial (medial tibial stress syndrome or MTSS)
about, 182–83
defining, 190
risk factors, 187
treating, 187–88
Shoes. *See also* Pronation and underpronation (supination)
for Achilles tendonitis, 162
Achilles tendonitis and, 160, 162
assessing condition of, 161
for barefoot running, 129–32
barefoot running and, 120–22, 123

buying (and trying on), 26–27, 161–62, 179
components and terms, 28–29
foot-related problems guide, 162
for half-marathons, 215
for high arches, 162
injury prevention and, 159–62
long runs and, 224
for low arches, 162
mileage on, 20, 37, 160, 161
minimalist, 131–32
for normal feet, 162
orthotics for, 31, 124, 129–30, 132, 172, 179, 189
plantar fasciitis and, 160–61
for post-stress fractures, 162
proprioception decrease from, 121
pushup test, 179
ramp angle, 122, 131
socks and, 32, 224, 260–61
sole composition and structure, 29
types of, 27–28
wearing and caring for, 30–31
when to buy, 20
Side stitches, 190–91
Social benefits of running, 9
Socializing, marathons and, 242–43
Socks, 32, 224, 260–61
Speed, 101–17
about: overview of, 101
downhill running and, 85–86
focusing on, precaution, 70
footstrikes and, 79–80
running form and, 74
stride and, 81–82
Speed work
adding, 102–4
beginner and novice runners, 113–14
cool-down routine, 112
experienced runners, 115–17
fartlek workouts, 106–7, 114, 115

Speed work—*continued*
  guidelines, 104–5
  hill repeats, 105–6
  interval workouts, 108–11
  mental edge from, 103
  risks and benefits, 102–4
  striders (pickups), 107–8
  tempo runs, 108
  warm-up routine, 111–12
Sports physician, selecting, 167–68
Stair-climbers, 91–92
Stance phase, 165–67
Starting out, 57–71. *See also*
  Stretching; Success tips
  beginner run/walk schedule, 59
  building base, 21–22, 68
  general guidelines, 58–60
  incrementally and gradually,
    18–19, 68–70
  mistakes to avoid, 22–24, 70–71
  precautions, 60–62
  10 percent rule, 69
  working with personal trainers, 67
Stepper machines, 91–92
Strassburg Sock®, 179
Stretching. *See also* Yoga
  after half-marathons, 217
  after marathons, 244
  avoiding overstretching, 164
  cool-down routine, 112
  fundamentals, 63–64
  importance of, 23, 63
  for injury prevention, 163–64
  Magic Six, Plus Two, 163–64
  muscle-specific stretches, 64–66
  warm-up routine, 111–12
Stride, 81–82, 139
Striders (pickups), 107–8
Style and mechanics. *See* Mechanics
  of running
Success tips, 11–24. *See also* Starting
  out
  about: overview of, 11

avoiding mistakes, 22–24, 70–71
choosing/sticking with program,
  16–19
commitment tools, 13–14
establishing foundation,
  19–22
making runs fun and convenient,
  17–18
runner's log and, 20–21, 35–38,
  272. *See also* Notebook
  (journal)
Supination. *See* Pronation and
  underpronation (supination)
Supplemental energy sources (gels,
  bars, etc.), 203, 226, 237, 242
Support wear, 32–33, 261. *See also*
  Shoes
Sweat rate, 44–46, 48
Swimming, 90
Swing phase, 165–66, 167

Tapering, 68–69, 114, 196, 206, 233.
  See also Reverse taper
Tempo runs, 108
10K Races
  about: overview of, 205
  after the race, 208–9
  mileage buildup for, 206–7
  next race after, 208–9
  running, 208
Time for running. *See also* Starting
  out
  choosing/sticking with program,
    16–19
  commitment tools, 13–14
  as excuse for not running, 2
  finding/making, 4, 12–13, 16–17
Training effect, 7
Travel and running
  lodging considerations, 270–71
  marathons, 236–39, 276
  planning for safety, 272–75
  racing, 275

seeing sights, 271–72
on vacation, 269–72
Treadmills, 266–69

Ultra-running
  defined, 248
  events, 249
  online resources, 283
  organizations, 248–49
  other preparations, 251
  physical preparation, 250–51
  training for ultra-runs, 249–51
  websites, 248
Uphill running, 85

Vacation, running and. *See* Travel
  and running
Visualization, 141, 165, 213, 229,
  232–33, 241
Vomiting, 184–85

Walls, climbing, 92
Warm-up routine, 111–12
Watches, 33–34
Water activities, 90–91
Water and hydration
  before, during, after run, 47, 48,
    49, 50
  body weight and, 45
  FAQs, 48, 49, 50–51
  for 5Ks, 197–98
  general guidelines, 61
  hot weather and, 262
  hyponatremia and, 49, 61, 198, 262
  importance of, 41, 44
  for long runs, 212–13, 225
  for running less than 60 minutes,
    22
  for running more than 60 minutes,
    34, 45
  speeding recovery, 264
  sports drinks, 34, 49, 61, 212–13
  sweat rate and, 44–46

Water bottles, 34
Weight
    before and after running, 45
    weight-conditioning program
        and, 99
Weight training
    about: overview of, 87
    for abs and back, 98–99
    benefits of, 92–94
    bent-over row, 96–97
    biceps curl, 96
    body weight and, 99
    front raise, 96
    guidelines, 94–95, 99–100
    leg curls, 97
    leg extensions, 97
    lower body exercises, 97
    lunges, 97
    pelvic tilt, 98
    practical training, 94–95
    repetitions (reps), 95
    running before, 100
    shoulder press, 96
    triceps kickback, 96
    types of weights, 95
    upper body exercises, 96–97
    upper body vs. lower body, 94
    using weights, 95
Women (and girls) and running,
    253–57
    about: overview of, 253
    comparing men and women,
        254–55
    female athlete triad, 54–55
    iron-deficiency anemia and,
        55–56
    menopause and, 256
    menstruation and, 255
    nutrition considerations,
        53–56
    osteoporosis and, 54, 93, 124, 255,
        256
    safety tips, 257

Year-round running, 259–76
    about: overview of, 259
    cold weather strategies, 260–61
    hot weather strategies, 262–65
    indoor running, 265–66
    treadmills for, 266–69
    vacation, travel and, 269–75
Yoga, 148–53
    Anusara® Yoga, 152
    Ashtanga Yoga, 151
    Baptiste Power Vinyasa Yoga®, 152
    benefits of, 148–50, 153
    Bikram Yoga®, 151
    finding your style, 150–52
    Indian styles, 151
    inward focus of, 152–53
    Iyengar Yoga®, 151
    Jivamukti Yoga®, 152
    OM Yoga, 152
    Sivananda® Yoga, 151
    United States styles, 152

We Have EVERYTHING® on Anything!

With more than 19 million copies sold, the Everything® series has become one of America's favorite resources for solving problems, learning new skills, and organizing lives. Our brand is not only recognizable—it's also welcomed.

The series is a hand-in-hand partner for people who are ready to tackle new subjects—like you!

For more information on the Everything® series, please visit *www.adamsmedia.com*

The Everything® list spans a wide range of subjects, with more than 500 titles covering 25 different categories:

Business	History	Reference
Careers	Home Improvement	Religion
Children's Storybooks	Everything Kids	Self-Help
Computers	Languages	Sports & Fitness
Cooking	Music	Travel
Crafts and Hobbies	New Age	Wedding
Education/Schools	Parenting	Writing
Games and Puzzles	Personal Finance	
Health	Pets	